AN INSIGHT BOOK

$N = 1$

Experimental Studies of Single Cases

An Enduring Problem in Psychology

Edited by
P. O. DAVIDSON
and
C. G. COSTELLO
Department of Psychology, University of Calgary

VAN NOSTRAND REINHOLD COMPANY
NEW YORK CINCINNATI TORONTO LONDON MELBOURNE

To M. B. Shapiro

Van Nostrand Reinhold Company Regional Offices:
Cincinnati, New York, Chicago, Millbrae, Dallas

Van Nostrand Reinhold Company Foreign Offices:
London, Toronto, Melbourne

Published by Van Nostrand Reinhold Company
450 West 33rd Street, New York, N. Y. 10001

Published simultaneously in Canada by
D. Van Nostrand Company (Canada), Ltd.

15 14 13 12 11 10 9 8 7 6 5 4 3 2 1

Preface

The generally useful distinction in science between observational and experimental studies has created some unnecessary but enduring problems for psychologists.

Because most experimental studies are based on group comparisons, many psychologists who are experimentally oriented believe that the single case cannot be used appropriately for purposes of fundamental research. At the same time, many clinical psychologists have been led to believe that the experimental method can make no useful contribution to their understanding of the unique problems of an individual case. Consequently, a split has often occurred between the clinicians and the experimentalists in psychology where each has tended to go his separate way in pursuing knowledge about human behavior.

In recent years some tentative bridges have been built across the gap separating the experimentalist and the clinician. The readings in this book represent some examples of one bridge of this kind. The studies presented differ in their theoretical orientation, the methods they use, the degree of experimental sophistication involved, and the extent of their success, but they all share in common an interest in applying experimental methods to the study of the individual case.

Some controversies about the rationale of this approach are discussed briefly in some of the articles and several methods of approach are described. While it is fairly easy to describe the experimental method in broad outline it is not so easy to put into practice. If the problems of abnormal psychology were easily susceptible to experimental inquiry the field would undoubtedly be more advanced than it is. The majority of the papers chosen for this book were therefore selected to give the reader specific examples of the problems and successes of this approach in dealing with actual cases.

The experimental study of the individual case as represented by these papers will—it is hoped—stimulate a greater interest in research in many clinicians and stimulate a greater interest in tackling unique clinical problems in many experimentalists.

Good examples of the application of experimental procedures are available in most areas of psychology except clinical psychology. For this reason all students and instructors in psychology may find this a valuable source book. Because of the immediate relevance of these methods in the clinical area this book will be of value to all mental health workers.

P. O. D.
C. G. C.

Contents

PREFACE iii

Part I—RATIONALE AND METHOD

1. EXPERIMENTAL METHOD IN THE PSYCHOLOGICAL DESCRIPTION OF THE INDIVIDUAL PSYCHIATRIC PATIENT 3
   M. B. Shapiro
2. STATISTICAL INFERENCE AND THE SINGLE CASE IN CLINICAL DESIGN 26
   J. B. Chassan
3. STATISTICS FOR THE INVESTIGATION OF INDIVIDUAL CASES 46
   R. W. Payne and H. Gwynne Jones

Part II—APPLICATIONS IN ASSESSMENT OF BEHAVIOR

4. A BLIND ANALYSIS OF A CASE OF MULTIPLE PERSONALITY USING THE SEMANTIC DIFFERENTIAL 61
   Charles E. Osgood and Zella Luria
5. AN ILLUSTRATION OF THE USE OF REPERTORY GRID TECHNIQUE IN A CLINICAL SETTING 88
   Fay Fransella and B. Adams
6. AN EXPERIMENTAL INVESTIGATION OF DISORDERED MOTOR EXPRESSION IN A CATATONIC SCHIZOPHRENIC PATIENT 105
   H. R. Beech and R. C. Parboosingh
7. AN INVESTIGATION OF AN ABNORMALITY OF COGNITIVE FUNCTION IN A COOPERATIVE YOUNG PSYCHOTIC: AN EXAMPLE OF THE APPLICATION OF EXPERIMENTAL METHOD TO THE SINGLE CASE 113
   M. B. Shapiro and E. H. Nelson
8. SPEED OF FUNCTION AND EDUCATIONAL RETARDATION: THE PSYCHOLOGICAL AND PSYCHIATRIC INVESTIGATION OF AN INDIVIDUAL CASE 128
   A. T. Ravenette and L. A. Hersov
9. DEMONSTRATION OF A PSYCHOSOMATIC RELATIONSHIP 147
   Maryse Metcalfe

Part III—APPLICATIONS IN TREATMENT

10. A LABORATORY STUDY OF FEAR: THE CASE OF PETER 157
    Mary Cover Jones

11. The Investigation and Treatment of a Reading Disability in a Child of Normal Intelligence 166
Singrida S. Ancevich and R. W. Payne
12. The Measurement of Clinically Relevant Variables 175
M. B. Shapiro
13. A Case Study in a Behavioral Analysis of Psychotherapy 188
Edward J. Murray
14. Aversive Control of Self-Injurious Behavior in a Psychotic Boy 202
B. G. Tate and George S. Baroff
15. An Approach to the Evaluation of Drug Effect During Psychotherapy: A Double-Blind Study of a Single Case 214
Leopold Bellak and J. B. Chassan

Part I

Rationale and Method

In spite of some enduring misconceptions, the application of statistical and experimental approaches to the single case is both possible and desirable. This application can require, however, a combination of flexible ingenuity and critical discipline that is not easy to achieve. Specifically, it requires that the intuitive, insightful generation of hypotheses about a patient be combined with the systematic objective evaluation of these hypotheses. It is unfortunate that the separate training and practice of clinical and experimental psychologists give them little opportunity to successfully combine these skills.

Shapiro, in the first paper in Part I, discusses the similarities and differences between the usual clinical methods and the experimental method. He demonstrates both by arguments and examples the considerable merits of adopting the experimental approach to individual cases. Shapiro demonstrates that the experimental investigation of the single case may produce results superior to the clinical investigation of it.

Chassan, in his paper, demonstrates that the intensive study of the single case may at times provide more meaningful information than that obtained from the traditional experimental method of extensive study of large samples. Chassan points out that the extensive study of small groups of psychiatric patients may sometimes result in serious errors of inference which do not occur in intensive studies of single cases.

In the final paper in this part, Payne and Jones supply some simple statistical procedures especially useful for the single case study. Many of the hypotheses psychologists formulate about their patients are based on inferences derived from test scores and particularly from discrepancies in test scores. Payne and Jones show how these discrepancies can be evaluated statistically in order to justify the hypotheses derived from them.

1

Experimental Method in the Psychological Description of the Individual Psychiatric Patient*

M. B. SHAPIRO

I. DEFINITION OF THE ROLE OF THE CLINICAL PSYCHOLOGIST

The distinctive role of the clinical psychologist can only be defined in terms of those activities, in the clinic and the hospital, which no one but an academically trained psychologist could carry out. This means that the psychologist should bring into psychiatry methods, generalizations and data from experimental psychology. This point is made because clinical psychologists, in describing their work, often give the impression that they play a part which could be played by any intelligent layman who had read about mental disorder and was familiar with its actual manifestations.

This would look like a statement of the obvious to someone who has not worked in the clinical field. However, as soon as one begins to work in this field, one finds a variety of trends and practices which obscure the issue, and which result in the development of complex arguments.

This paper will discuss that part of clinical psychology which is concerned with the description of psychological function. This is the most widely practised part of clinical psychology.

---

* Reprinted from the *International Journal of Social Psychiatry*, 1957, Vol. 3, pp. 89–102, by permission of the author and the publisher.

II. RULES OF VALID PSYCHOLOGICAL DESCRIPTION

Experimental psychology has some definite advice to give on the methodology of psychological description. In the first place it advises us to use standardized methods. This means that we have to use standard repeatable situations, and standard repeatable methods of evaluating and quantifying responses to these situations. We are dealing here with the characteristics of a mental test.

The second requirement of experimental psychology is that of validation. Correlation is one of the main requirements of descriptive validity. The ascribing of any characteristic to an individual in the clinic must have implications for his behaviour outside. Otherwise the description is useless, and we commit what Spearman labelled a "faculty error."

The third requirement in psychological description is that of calibration. Once we have validated a certain method of describing a psychological characteristic, we need to know how much of it a subject possesses. The usual method of doing this is to give our test to a sample which is representative of the population which is relevant to our purpose. We can compare the score which any particular patient obtains on that test with the distribution of scores we obtained from our sample, and this indicates how much of the particular characteristic the patient has.

To summarize, we can say that we derive from academic psychology three requirements for adequate psychological description. They are those of standardization, validation, and calibration.

The foregoing may, to many psychologists, sound like a statement of the obvious. It is important, however, to remind ourselves of these three requirements because certain prominent trends in clinical psychology and psychiatry consist of making a virtue of ignoring and breaking the obvious rules.

III. INTUITIVE AND ARTISTIC METHODS

The most drastic way of breaking the rules consists of openly throwing them all overboard. That is done by those who claim that there is no place, for the time being at least, for science and experiment in clinical psychology, and that, therefore, the clinical psychologist leans mainly on his intuition, or that he practises an art. There is no argument that can get over the fact that the antiscientist must produce acceptable evidence that his methods work, and that he actually helps his patients. He should not expect to be taken seriously until he does so. This requirement is given added point by the fact that attempts to validate such approaches have, as Eysenck (*3*) has pointed out, produced poor results.

It would appear, from recent discussions within the British Psychological Society, that some psychologists try to deal with this challenge by cultivating a halo of authority on the basis of mere familiarity with the sufferings of the mentally ill. Some try to reinforce this authority by referring to the heavy responsibilities which the sufferings of their patients impose upon them. They use this authority to back the assertion that the phenomena of mental illnesses are too complex and too subtle to be objectively measured. Such an assertion can have little weight when we are not even in a position to point to a record of long and stubborn attempts to apply the methods of objective measurement.

IV. THE "FLEXIBLE" METHOD

In addition to those who make a virtue of casting aside openly the rules of scientific psychological description, there are those who adopt a more indirect approach. Two main variations of this have appeared. The first consists of using objective methods of measurement in a so-called "flexible" manner. A flexible approach is advocated because human nature is said to be too complex and subtle to be described by the use of rigid procedures. For example, in the case of intelligence testing, it has often been argued in recent discussions that it is necessary to alter the method of administering the test in order to suit the supposed needs of the patient. It is proposed that changes should be made arbitrarily, without any particular system, in any way that the psychologist thinks fit during the test. If one does this, one is in duty bound to cast aside the pretence of using a standardized validated test. The psychiatrist and social worker would then know exactly how much weight to place on the psychologist's results. They would not be misled by the apparent objectivity of the methods used.

Aside from breaking the rules of psychological measurement, this approach appears to be incorrect because it does not put pressure upon the clinical psychologist to acquire the right kind of skills. One of the most important skills that a clinical psychologist should have is that of obtaining a standard test result from the most difficult of patients. Two examples will illustrate this point.

The first example is concerned with a seven-year-old girl who would not co-operate properly with the writer during a test and was occasionally very aggressive, making quite strong but not very effective attempts to hit him. The child was suspected of being a mental defective, and therefore it was necessary to obtain as reliable an estimate as possible of the child's intelligence. The first session was spent with the child in the playroom without any result. The psychologist made a number of unsuccessful attempts to get the child to carry out instructions. In the second session the patient continued to be aggressive. As a last resort the psychologist threw one of the toys against the wall and smashed it. The child smiled and said: "Do it again." The psychologist asked the child to fetch him a toy to do this. The child did so and another toy was thrown against the wall. By bringing the toy to the psychologist she carried out an instruction for the first time. Play began to develop in which further instructions were given and carried out, until over the remainder of this and yet another session it was possible to administer the Terman-Merrill and obtain a clearly non-defective score.

A second example arising from the writer's experience is that of a young woman who would not talk, and about whom the question of mental deficiency was raised. She was presented with Raven's Matrices. For the first three-quarters of an hour the patient did not carry out any of the writer's requests. It was finally possible to persuade the patient to indicate with a slight movement of her finger which of a number of the multiple-choice items she though was correct. The patient produced a clearly non-defective score in this manner.

It is, of course, sometimes necessary to change the test procedure to obtain a test result. This does not mean that one should change the procedures in an arbitrary manner: e.g. by unsystematic alterations, the repetition of instructions, the extension of time limits, and the repetition of trials. It only means that one must at times introduce into the test procedure a systematic variation which produces, as nearly as the conditions will allow, a quantifiable and repeatable observation. An example of this will illustrate the point.

This example is based on an experience of Dr. R. W. Payne. He had tested a male G.P.I. and obtained a score indicating defective intelligence. Such a score, in relation to the patient's case history, indicated considerable intellectual deterioration. Dr. Payne felt that this indication might be seriously in error, because it seemed to him that the patient's intellectual condition fluctuated. The patient sometimes seemed to talk quite rationally and at other times he appeared to be clearly disordered. Dr. Payne then retested the patient on the Matrices in the following manner. He instructed the patient to make comments on the test items, and on the way he worked them out while he was doing the test. As soon as Dr. Payne thought that the patient was displaying disordered thinking he took the Matrices booklet away. He kept talking to the patient until it seemed that the patient was being rational again and then returned the book for the patient to continue the test as before. This procedure was continued until the test was finished. The patient now obtained an improved score. Payne now had evidence that the patient's intellectual efficiency fluctuated considerably, and he was therefore able to begin an investigation of the causes of this fluctuation and the degree to which it could be controlled to the patient's benefit.

We cannot discuss here the general implications of these last three examples for a theory of obtaining reliable test results from difficult patients. We cite them only to show that the clinical psychologist will neglect the development of important skills if he regards the mental test as a rough procedure which enables him to make subjective judgments about a patient's qualities.

V. THE ECLECTIC APPROACH

Another method of breaking the rules of objective measurement is that of adopting an apparently detached and eclectic attitude. This consists of pointing out that there are two forms of observation, quantitative and qualitative, and that while quantitative methods have their uses there are important qualitative observations to be made which cannot be quantified.

A good example of this approach is provided by R. Schafer (*12*). He points out on p. 17 that in response to the Wechsler Comprehension item "Why should we keep away from bad company?" each of the following responses would obtain a maximum score of two: "They have a terrible influence on our character and lead us into evil ways" and "I don't have much use for the concept of bad company, but we're supposed to believe that they will corrupt us." Schafer claims that the subject in this way communicates more "than he wittingly intends; *he also communicates more than can be scored.* Test responses, because they represent the subject's style of thinking, allow for inferences concerning predominant features of the character make-up." (Our [Shapiro's] italics.)

Is it really true that we have here an example of responses that cannot be scored? Let us look at the two responses again. The first response is consistent with a complete and exaggerated identification with current social morals. The second is consistent with the opposite. It would be relatively easy to devise a rating scale which quantified such extreme responses and which also quantified responses of an intermediate degree of conformity. It would also be possible to invent other items which were aimed at evoking similar responses, and they too could be quantified. Once we had done that, we would be faced with the two routine problems of psychological measurement. First of all, we would want to find how much consistency there was in social conformity responses from one kind of item to another, i.e. is there a factor of social conformity? If the evidence were consistent with such a factor we would go on to standardize our new test on sample representatives of the population we were interested in.

It seems that the essential fallacy in Schafer's argument is the assumption that qualitative and quantitative approaches are mutually exclusive, when in fact the two are complementary. Usually the most efficient way of investigating and making use of a qualitative observation is to quantify it, and the ability to do so is primarily a question of ingenuity and time.

It is recognized, of course, that the Wechsler Test, in its present form, has been made to serve one purpose: the measurement of cognitive efficiency. We have, therefore, no means of scoring those aspects of a subject's responses which throw light on his "character make-up." In these circumstances it is necessary for the psychologist to listen to his subject's responses and to take note of those aspects of the responses which are not measured by the test in its present form. In making clinical use of such observations the psychologist should be under no illusion about what he is doing. He is in fact using an unvalidated and unstandardized test. This is essentially what many so-called clinical observations are. He should, therefore, take steps to check such observations as carefully as his circumstances would allow. It is one thing to be forced by circumstances to use makeshift methods. It is quite another to make a virtue of doing so. One might object that this argument over-complicates what are in many cases obvious observations, and that such obvious observations are an important part of psychological description. Our own experience shows that even the most "obvious" observations are often contaminated by error and invalid inference. Two examples from our files will suffice to illustrate the point.

The first example has been described in greater detail elsewhere (*13*). The patient, a young adult male, was given a part of a newspaper to read out aloud during a ward round. When he had finished he was asked to say what he had read, and he could remember nothing. He was referred to the psychologist for a possible reading defect. He had already produced a well above average score on the Wechsler Intelligence test. Two reading comprehension tests, which were standardized on young children, were given to the patient. He obtained almost zero scores on both tests. The reading tests were then given to nine graduate psychologists in the department. Some of them obtained scores which were nearly as bad as those of the patient.

The clinician had evidently made a reliable observation when he found that the patient could not give the gist of a passage he had read aloud. The assumption that this ability was highly abnormal for an intelligent young adult was, however, erroneous since in fact it was not sufficiently abnormal to warrant a firm conclusion that the patient suffered from a reading defect.

A second example is that of a patient who was consistently judged by anyone who met him as being "very withdrawn." An investigation of his cognitive functions had revealed the fact that he was extremely slow in all cognitive tasks, though the level he could reach in his own time might be very high. One theory put up to explain this finding was that the presence of the psychologist disturbed him. To check this notion, the patient was tested under two conditions: with the psychologist present and the psychologist absent. The patient, as before, was very slow when the psychologist was present, but he was even worse when the psychologist was absent. Two further experiments confirmed this finding.

These results had two effects. They threw doubt on the idea that the reason why the patient was slow was because he found the psychologist's presence disturbing. In fact, it seemed as if the patient needed the presence of the psychologist to maintain his already poor rate of work. In the second place, one now could argue that the subjective impression that the patient was withdrawn, no matter how reliable in itself, did not mean that the patient did not react to social stimulation. In fact, one might argue from the data we had gathered that the patient was dependent on social stimulation for the maintenance of his poor rate of performance.

It is not being advocated here that the psychologist must take no notice of what the patient says and does, or that the psychologist may not have "hunches" which are quite valid, but which are difficult to make explicit. The argument merely is that the psychologist should be distinguished by the fact that he consistently aims at objectifying his conceptions and by the fact that he is skilled at doing this.

In addition, the argument which has been developed so far does not mean that the psychologist should refuse to give an opinion when time and opportunity prevent him from validating his theories about a patient. Decisions have to be made, and they frequently have to be made on the basis of opinions. It is one thing, however, to know that your opinion is largely an untested hypothesis; that it is the hypothesis which, in the light of all the available clinical and psychometric data, you think is most likely to prove correct. It is quite another thing to claim that there is a special virtue in utilizing such untested opinions, to give them an aura of respectability by calling the practice "clinical method," or "the qualitative approach." To do this ensures that we stultify the development of objective psychological knowledge in the clinic. All we will continue to achieve is the ambiguous mass of anecdote which constitutes a large part of contemporary psychiatry and clinical psychology.

VI. THE LIMITATIONS OF OBJECTIVE METHODS

Objective methods of psychological description have undoubted limitations. The first of these limitations arises out of the fact that measurement is always in error to a more or less extent. One of the main virtues of objective measurement is that it gives you a more accurate idea of how much you might be in error. For example, a test with a reliability of .9, a standard deviation of 16 and a mean of 100 will have a standard error of measurement of about 5 points of I.Q. This means, for example, that one-third of the measurements of an individual will differ by 10 points or more from his true test measure. (We assume, of course, that the influence of practice has been ruled out.) The clinical psychologist usually does not know where exactly on the band of error the true score is likely to be.

Unreliability, of course, is not the only source of error in measurement. We have error which arises out of the limited validity of many of our measures and the error which arises out of the faulty calibration of our tests. It is one thing to say that one calibrates a test by giving it to a representative sample of a defined population. It is quite another thing to find such a sample. Thus the objective clinical psychologist who uses objective methods is always haunted by the handmaiden of measurement: error. One of his main preoccupations becomes that of finding methods of combating error. This, of course, is a preoccupation in every applied science.

Aside from the limitation of error, we have the fact that the making of good tests is a time-consuming and expensive business. It took a large team of workers nine years to make and standardize the Terman Merrill Binet. Furthermore, the present undeveloped state of clinical psychology as a systematized science means that there is a limit to the number of useful tests which can at the present time be developed. These considerations mean that we cannot look forward to the rapid provision of a wide range of useful tests.

VII. EXPERIMENTAL METHOD

It would seem from the foregoing discussion that the psychologist faces a dilemma. On the one hand he needs to use objective methods. On the other hand he has only a few validated and standardized measures at his disposal, and the few he has are prone to error.

It would seem that aside from pushing forward our fundamental research as hard as we can, this dilemma can only be dealt with, not by abandoning scientific method, but rather by its continuous and persistent application. This aim is facilitated by adding a fourth rule to our three rules of psychological description, a rule which, it seems, was first formulated in relation to clinical psychology by Goldstein, (*4*) though he has not practised it in the manner to be discussed in this paper. According to this rule, it is possible to test a theory about an individual's behaviour by predicting from such a theory how his behaviour will vary from one circumstance to another. In making such a prediction one is, of course, assisted by the use of standardized tests; but these are not always necessary.

As illustrations of this application of our fourth rule, we can refer back to two of the examples which we gave above. In the case of the G.P.I. patient, the theory was tested that the patient did not suffer from a stable intellectual impairment but from a fluctuating one. This was done by retesting the patient only while there was no indication of thought disorder. In the case of the "withdrawn" patient, the theory that the patient did not react to social stimulation was tested by making the patient do the test under two conditions: with the psychologist present and absent.

Goldstein and Scheerer (*5*) have contrasted this method with psychometric method. They call their method a qualitative method, and psychometric method a quantitative one. In their view, the former has considerable advantages over the latter. One of their examples is a patient with an apparent alexia. Such a patient would obtain a zero score on conventional reading for comprehension test. When, however, a frame is placed around the word, the word is correctly read.

Goldstein and Scheerer go on to imply that the psychometrist would come to a false conclusion that the patient had no reading ability, while the so-called qualitative psychologist would establish that the capacity to read was still present. This argument is based on two misconceptions. The first misconception is that this example demonstrates the mutual exclusiveness of the quantitative and qualitative aspect of psychological observation. We are merely dealing here with two extreme scores: zero and maximum. Without the frame the patient obtains a zero score for reading the words, and with the frame he obtains a maximum score.

The second misconception is that the fact that the patient can read with the frame completely invalidates the zero score he obtained by the more conventional test. The objective psychologist who obtains a zero score from a brain-damaged patient does not immediately conclude that the patient cannot read under any circumstances. This itself is an hypothesis that needs to be tested. He would know that a variety of conditions might restore, at least temporarily, a brain-damaged patient's ability to read. Among such conditions are an injection of sodium amytal and a loud continuous noise, as well as the frame. If it were relevant to the patient's diagnosis, treatment, or disposal, he might then test the patient's ability to read under these various conditions. It seems that Goldstein and Scheerer, in order to make their point, have had to direct their fire at the worst kind of clinical psychologist: the clinical psychologist who does not know any clinical psychology.

These criticisms must not, however, blind us to the importance of their contribution. This consists of indicating how a generalization about a single individual can be tested by observing the systematic variation of his behaviour with changes in conditions. *This enables us to reduce the error of the conclusions we come to, and to make discoveries about the mode of psychological function of our patients without waiting for leads from fundamental research.* Both these points are illustrated by the experiment quoted above: the one on the G.P.I. patient and the other on the "withdrawn" patient.

In the case of the G.P.I. patient, the first very low score on the Matrices would have been seriously in error, and the demonstration of the fact that it fluctuated according to changes in the patient's state, reduced the error of the estimate of his intelligence. Payne was able to make this determination without waiting for fundamental research on the effects of fluctuating thought disorder on intelligence test performance.

In the case of the "withdrawn" patient, it was possible to make observations of the effects of social stimulation on a patient's test performance without waiting for fundamental research to be done in this field. The results were at least definite enough to throw doubts on the validity of the inference that the patient did not require social stimulation.

VIII. MAIN CHARACTERISTICS OF THE EXPERIMENTAL METHOD

In practice it is not sufficient to say that a descriptive generalization about a patient can be validated by the use of experimental method on a single case. In fact, the arrival at the point of a validated generalization which has implications for the patient concerned involves some sophistication of method and theory. If we are to achieve such sophistication, and communicate it to others, it is necessary to make explicit the main principles of scientific clinical investigation and indicate the lines along which these principles should be applied.

The aim of the descriptive investigation should usually be that of the explanation of a given observation. This involves three phases. The first is the exact formulation of the observation which is to be explained. The second phase is the formulation of testable explanation of the observation. The third phase is the testing of propositions which have been rigorously deduced from the explanation.

IX. THE SELECTION OF AN OBSERVATION FOR INVESTIGATION

The observation which is investigated is usually, in our practice so far, an abnormality of psychological function. This abnormality may be a psychiatric symptom, it may be a feature that appears in the course of a test, or it may be a discrepancy between two test results. The kind of observation one chooses to investigate will depend on a number of considerations, such as its actual importance for the patient's adjustment, its amenability to exact investigation, and the amount of relevant scientific information known to be available.

In every case the strict statistical notion of abnormality is implied: in terms of the distribution of the characteristic concerned in the normal population. Control data are, therefore, necessary. Such data can take various forms: (i) Published control data such as those of a standardized test and which require no additional treatment. (ii) Data which require further treatment. For example, if there is a discrepancy between two test results we can, if we know the intercorrelation and the means and standard deviations of the two tests, make an estimate of the abnormality of the difference by applying the formula for the standard deviation of difference. (*11*) (iii) Data which one collects oneself. For example, a seven-year-old patient produced a drawing of a house, which appeared to be highly abnormal. The psychologist concerned—Mrs. Margaret Evans—asked the local school to obtain drawings of a house from all its seven-year-olds, and the impression of the abnormality of the drawing was confirmed. (iv) Using a single control. For example, in one of our cases we wished to investigate the learning and retention processes of a patient who had resisted attempts to teach him to read. To begin with we wanted to find out which of these processes was most likely to be abnormal. In order to obtain an indication of this, we gave learning and retention tests to the patient, and to another patient who was of the same age and I.Q. as our first patient, but who was a good reader. In each of the tests we had a number of observations for each subject and so we were able to apply tests of significance to the distribution obtained. We found that our patient differed significantly from the control in learning but not in retention. This result indicated that the abnormality lay in the learning processes and not in retention, a finding which was made conclusive by now giving the learning tests to other readers and non-readers of the same age and I.Q. (v) An "obvious" abnormality, in estimating which one implicitly uses as a control one's own and one's colleagues' experience. The risks of this procedure can be very great, as is shown by the example of the intelligent young man described above, who was apparently unable to understand material which he read aloud, but who was finally shown to share this difficulty with normal subjects.

X. THE SELECTION OF EXPLANATIONS

The kind of explanation one chooses to investigate depends on at least the following considerations:

(i) The amount of psychometric and clinical data for which the explanation appears to account and the range of its implications for the subject's behaviour. The most adequate explanation would in fact be the "opinion" one would advance if one did not have the time to investigate the case any further.

(ii) The implications for the treatment and disposal of the case. For example, the establishment of a general disability in the handling of spatial relations might have little importance for a student of languages but considerable importance for an engineer.

(iii) The case of testing an hypothesis. Before embarking on a relatively complex investigation, one might be inclined to get a relatively unimportant hypothesis out of the way, if it could be checked with a simple and short test.

(iv) The help one can obtain from general and clinical psychology in the development and testing of the hypotheses concerned. For example, the fact that a patient's speed of cognitive work shows an abnormal decrease with increase of difficulty level, suggests that the Yerkes-Dodson law might be operating. Experimental work concerning this law might suggest testable hypotheses to explain the difficulty.

This last consideration touches on one of the main problems in clinical psychology: the need to systematize, for its own purpose, the findings of general and experimental psychology. It should be noted that data and generalizations concerning such topics as the organization of human ability, the learning processes, child development, perception and thinking, are not yet being systematically applied in the clinical field. This is not because clinical psychologists have tried them out and found them wanting: but because on *a priori* grounds they have not yet considered it possible to use them.

The first hypothesis which must be considered as a matter of routine is that the observation is unreliable or an artefact of inappropriate standardization of the measure. An example of this is found in an investigation by J. G. Ingham. One of his patients produced a very low score on Thurstone's Primary Mental Abilities test and a high score on Raven's Matrices. As the first test is speeded and the second is not, this result seemed to throw light on the patient's reported scholastic backwardness. Before investigating this further, Ingham gave the two tests to the patient's classmates and found that they, too, did worse on the P.M.A. than the Matrices. This indicated that the P.M.A. was more difficult than the Matrices for the London children, and not that the patient's scholastic backwardness was due to slowness of cognitive function.

Finally, it should be remembered that there can be many more than one determinant of a given abnormality. Explanations are, therefore, rarely mutually exclusive.

XI. METHODS OF TESTING AN HYPOTHESIS

Methods of testing an hypothesis are limited only by the actual range of possible observations of psychological phenomena. At the one extreme an hypothesis may be tested by bringing an abnormality under direct experimental control. For example, Payne (*10*) carried out an experiment which showed that a certain patient's highly abnormal rambling speech occurred only when he was talking to somebody else but not when he had to formulate answers to questions while he was alone. On the other hand, we have an example provided by Metcalfe, (*7*)* who tested the

* See Reading 9, this book.—EDS.

hypothesis that a patient's asthmatic attacks were connected with the mother, by keeping a record of all the attacks and all the patient's main activities. The outcome showed a highly significant connection between meetings with the mother and attacks of asthma.

It is often difficult to decide which is the best hypothesis to test, to be sure that one has advanced an explanation which best accounts for one's data, and that one has not in fact committed some grave error of reasoning or overlooked some important fact. While it is necessary to be as careful and as rigorous as possible, one learns not to worry too much about these considerations. What matters most is that the observations are built up in some kind of systematic manner. Muddle and oversight may serve to slow one up, but the character of the data, as it accumulates about a patient, tends to assert itself if one is always ready to drop one's preconceptions and to generalize from the facts as one finds them.

It should be borne in mind that one can test an hypothesis by using the patient as his own control. Zubin (*15*) gives an example of this method in his investigation of the effects of E.C.T. on a patient's learning process. By making a large number of observations under each of the relevant different conditions, it is possible to apply tests of significance to the distributions obtained under the two conditions. Thus, if we had reason to expect that a patient's average time per item would increase with a given change in conditions, and in fact it falls significantly, then we can at least say that we have a reliable change of performance which is contrary to expectation. Work, however, still needs to be done on the application of sampling theory to tests of a null hypothesis on the single case, because the observations in a single case are not strictly independent. We now have to consider the general implications of the approach for clinical psychology.

XII. CLINICAL RESEARCH

The carrying out of an experimental descriptive investigation to a relatively definite and useful conclusion is usually very difficult and time-consuming. Reference to papers by Payne, (*10*)

Jones (*6*) and Bartlett and Shapiro (*1*) will provide an indication of this. Investigations of this kind make as much demand for originality and precision of thinking as does the best fundamental research. The result is that a clinical psychologist will rarely be able, in addition to his other work, to conduct more than one or two experimental investigations at a time. In fact, this kind of work is a form of research and perhaps the most appropriate name for it is "clinical research."

The main aim of clinical research is the diagnosis, treatment, and adjustment of the patient on whom the research is done. This is different from other research which seeks for information which does not benefit those patients who take part. This does not mean that much of clinical research will not have implications beyond the patient concerned; but that will only be coincidental.

Clinical research should have two outcomes. The first outcome of research should be the provision of information on ways in which already validated and standardized techniques can be applied in the clinical field. For example, the Wechsler-Bellevue Test of Intelligence was prepared as a cognitive test with an equivalent form; two scales—the Verbal and Performance Scales; and a variety of subtests. The content of these scales and tests varies in different ways, e.g. the relative familiarity as to the subject, in the relative role of speed, and in verbal and spatial content. We need to investigate the clinical use, if any, of these different aspects of the test. The manual does not provide any information. An illustrative example is a finding by Mrs. Berenice Krikler. When first tested with the Wechsler-Bellevue, the patient concerned produced a Verbal I.Q. of 132 and a Performance I.Q. of 101. The difference was significant at less than the .001 level (for method calculation see [*11*] *). When retested with Form II months later, the discrepancy was reduced to 7 points. At the same time, however, some new test material again provoked a low score, which in turn improved on second test with an equivalent form. This led to the generalization that the patient was sometimes very badly affected by new situations. We now not only have some useful information about the patient but we have

* See Reading 3, this book.—EDS.

learnt a new use for some tests with equivalent forms. They can be used to measure the effects of an unfamiliar situation upon cognitive performance.

A second outcome of clinical research is that we should be able to investigate the usefulness of the method of using the patient as his own control, when the sole aim is the successful treatment and adjustment of the patient concerned. The question arises whether control data of the traditional kind is required at all if one can always predict accurately the patient's behaviour in different situations.

The extensive application of the physical sciences has depended upon the intensive development of applied research. It took the experimental activities of a Marconi for us to reap the benefits of the fundamental research of Hertz. It seems that we need to establish a tradition and a literature of clinical research. Gradually, as our experience develops, and as we become able to systematize and use the relevant parts of general and abnormal psychology, we should be able increasingly to routinize our approach to patients and to develop standard techniques of testing certain hypotheses. The number of patients that the psychologist can effectively help should gradually increase.

XIII. THE EFFECTS OF THIS APPROACH ON ROUTINE WORK

1. The Discarding of Invalid or Unvalidated Procedures

We have now to consider the effect of this approach on our work with the majority of our patients. In the first place it means that we cannot use routinely unvalidated and unstandardized procedures for the purpose of arriving at conclusions about a patient. Most of the popular projective tests and many tests of brain damage appear to fall into this category.

2. Bridging the Gap between General and Clinical Psychology

The discarding of non-valid or unvalidated procedures means that many psychologists can be released from the operation of time-consuming batteries of tests. They can instead face up to the actual psychological problems presented by psychiatric patients. This involves finding out whether general and experimental psychology have anything to offer in the way of explanation of the patient's disorders, and whether this explanation gives any leads for further investigation, treatment, and disposal of the patient. Relatively definite answers to such questions, whether they be positive or negative in outcome, involve, aside from actual experimentation with the patient, a systematic investigation of the experimental literature. For example, one of the implications of the relative inconstancy of the I.Q. (*2*) is that a child may be relatively bright when he is young and lose his intellectual superiority as he becomes older. Such a child's parents and teachers might, therefore, be wrong in ascribing his subsequent drop in attainment to some kind of personality defect. The drop may have been due to biological factors.

Another example is the well-known finding of May and Hartshorne, (*8*) that there is a low correlation between different tests of honesty in children. The honesty of a child seems to depend more on specific factors like the presence or absence of certain friends, the kind of motive involved, and the particular person who happens to be his teacher.

A third example is the finding reported by Murphy *et al.* (*9*) (p. 464), that aggression and sympathy in young children tend to be correlated. The more aggressive child tends also to be the more sympathetic one.

The experimental literature is quite well stocked with facts and generalizations which are waiting to be systematized in relation to the problems of clinical psychology. It would therefore seem, to be far more useful, in relation to any given case, to put at the psychiatrist's disposal the outcome of eight hours of relevant study of the experimental literature, than to spend the same time on a battery of unvalidated or invalid tests.

3. *Limited Investigations*

We should be willing to conduct investigations of a limited character directed at answering questions which are clinically relevant. There may be no test for deciding whether a patient has an anxiety neurosis, but at least one can find out what behaviour characteristics the psychiatrist thinks such a patient should have and try to measure them objectively. An experiment by Mrs. Metcalfe will illustrate the point.

The patient concerned had a tic. It was believed that the tic was due to stress. The psychiatrist defined what he meant by a stress or lack of stress for this patient. The patient was then placed in both a stressed and unstressed situation and the frequency of tics in each type of situation recorded. The patient in fact produced the tic far more frequently in the relaxed situation than he did in the stressed situation.

The use of limited experimentation often arouses strong opposition from clinical psychologists. For purpose of illustration let us again consider the case of the patient who was tested once with the psychologist present and once with the psychologist absent. This observation was made only three times. In the first place, one could argue that three occasions were not enough. His improved performances in the presence of the psychologist might have been accidental. If we had carried out further experiments the consistency of the findings might have disappeared.

In the second place, if the observation had been reliable, it may still have had no relation whatever to the social aspects of the situation. Perhaps *any* interrupting stimulus, such as a flickering light or a continuous sound, might have disinhibited our subject, and speeded him up.

Finally, one might argue that, in any case, control data were necessary before coming to any conclusions. How do we know that a control group of normal subjects, when tested on their own, would not have slowed down more than our patient and that, therefore, the truth was that our patient was *relatively* unreactive to social stimulation?

The implications of criticisms of this kind are that the scientific clinical psychologist should: (i) establish unequivocally the reliability of every observation; (ii) test all possible alternative explanations; and (iii) collect all relevant control data.

The reply to this argument is that the clinical psychologist must give opinions. His opinions are, in fact, the hypotheses which he thinks to be the most likely ones in the light of all the clinical and psychometric evidence, and his knowledge of psychology. As far as possible he bases these opinions on objective and repeatable observations. He gives more weight to these. It is better to know that a patient produces, say, an average score under one condition of testing and a very much below average score under another condition of testing, than to have one single apparently reliable score which places the patient as being very inferior or as being average.

In the last analysis, all procedures have to be subject to actuarial investigation. We need to do appropriate follow-up studies in which we measure relative efficiency of different approaches. We can, however, only carry out such studies when we have become skilled in the application of experimental method.

XIV. PART-WHOLE RELATIONS

One of the main implications of this approach is that the meticulous and detailed experimental investigation of an aspect of abnormal psychological function will yield results which have important implications for a psychiatric patient's psychological adjustment. This implies that various aspects of psychological function interact with each other and that, therefore, the understanding of one aspect of psychological function should throw light on other aspects. Although this assumption is a plausible one, it needs itself to be investigated and tested.

Psychologists are often harassed by the fear that close attention to detail will not produce important results. They are apparently so influenced by arbitrary conceptions concerning the qualitative uniqueness of each act of human behaviour that they are afraid of becoming lost among trivialities if they undertake an experimental investigation.

XV. EXPERIMENTAL METHOD AND THE NEEDS OF THE PATIENT

The conclusion from this discussion is that the main role of the clinical psychologist should be to develop stubbornly and persistently his contribution to psychiatry as an experimental psychologist. His aim in doing this is not merely to comply in a ritualistic manner with the rules of science. The aim is the welfare of the patient. It is to the interests of the patient that the ideas the psychologist has about the patient should be correct, and that the psychologist should be skilled in formulating ideas derived from his science and establishing their validity. It seems to be incorrect to maintain that there is a divorce between the urgent needs of the psychiatric patient and the fulfilment of the most rigorous requirements of scientific method. On the contrary, there can, once we have decided to serve the patient's needs, be a complete identity of the interests of the patient with the most rigorous requirements of science.

REFERENCES

1. BARTLETT, D., and SHAPIRO, M. B. Investigation and treatment of a reading disability in a dull child with severe psychiatric disturbances. *Brit. J. educ. Psychol.*, November, 1956, vol. XXVI, part III, 180–190.
2. CLARKE, A. D. B., and CLARKE, A. M. How constant is the I.Q.? *Lancet,* 1953, 877–894.
3. EYSENCK, H. J. *The Scientific Study of Personality*. London: Kegan Paul, 1952.
4. GOLDSTEIN, K. *The Organism*. New York: American Book Co. (American Psychology Series), 1939.
5. GOLDSTEIN, K., and SCHEERER, M. Abstract and concrete behaviour. *Psychol. Monog.*, 1941, vol. 53, no. 2.
6. JONES, H. G. The application of conditioning and learning techniques to the treatment of a psychiatric patient. *J. abnorm. soc. Psychol.*, 1956, vol. 52, 414–419.
7. METCALFE, M. Demonstration of a psychosomatic relationship. *Brit. J. med. Psychol.*, 1956, vol. XXIX, 1, 63–66.
8. MAY, M., and HARTSHORNE, H. *Studies in the Nature of Character. Book 2: Statistical Methods and Results.* London: Macmillan Co., 1930.
9. MURPHY, G., MURPHY, L. B., and NEWCOMB, T. M. *Experimental Social Psychology*. New York: Harper, 1937.
10. PAYNE, R. W. The role of the clinical psychologist at the Institute of Psychiatry. *Revue de Psychologie appliquée* (Revue Trimestrielle), July, 1953, tome 3, no. 3, 150–160.
11. PAYNE, R. W., and JONES, H. G. Statistics for the investigation of individual cases. *J. clin. Psychol.* 1957, 13, 115–121.
12. SCHAFER, R. *The Clinical Application of Psychological Tests.* New York: Menninger Foundation, Series 6, Internat. Univ. Press, 1948.

13. SHAPIRO, M. B. An experimental approach to diagnostic psychological testing. *J. ment. Sci.,* 1951, vol. 97, no. 408, 748–764.
14. SHAPIRO, M. B., and NELSON, E. H. An investigation of an abnormality of cognitive function in a co-operative young psychotic: an example of the application of the experimental method to the single case. *J. clin. Psychol.,* 1955, vol. 11, no. 4, 344–351.
15. ZUBIN, J. Objective studies of disordered persons. (In T. G. Andrew's *Methods in Psychology*. London: J. Wiley and Sons, 1948.)

2

Statistical Inference and the Single Case in Clinical Design*

J. B. CHASSAN

The advent of the tranquilizers in the last few years has given rise to a tremendous outpouring of research effort in clinical psychiatry and the behavioral sciences in general. Contributors to this effort have come from a number of diverse subject-matter backgrounds and disciplines. Yet despite this great expenditure of research energy, comparatively little progress has been made thus far in at least one very important area. This is the area of the design of clinical studies—in particular, the design of studies involving the use of tranquilizers in the setting of the mental hospital. In this paper, I shall present certain advantages of the intensive statistical study of the individual patient, as affording information with operational significance which cannot possibly be achieved otherwise.

While some of the difficulty in designing clinical studies in the mental hospital may inhere in the subject matter itself, a major obstacle, upon critical examination, seems to be an attitude, on the part of many investigators, of apparently unquestioning acceptance of certain conceptions and misconceptions about experimental design and related statistical methodology. It is unfortunate that some of these attitudes and procedures have become so ingrained in the minds of many investigators that they mistakenly consider one or another of them as the whole of scientific method, or as the whole of the statistical aspect of scientific method, and proceed to construct experimental designs in deference to various of these methodological deities with overpowering odds against obtaining any operationally usable data from them, or against using otherwise useful data in an operationally meaningful way.

---

* Reprinted from *Psychiatry,* 1960, Vol. 23, pp. 173–184, by permission of the author and the publisher.

One of the basic limitations under which clinical research often has to be performed is the relatively small number of patients available for a given study, particularly with respect to the large number of variables which may, at least in theory, affect behavior or symptomatology. This limitation can come about in any of a number of ways: administrative difficulties, medical counterindications, limited financial resources, a shortage of personnel, and, last but not least, the small number of patients fulfilling a set of criteria for selection in a given institution.

Suppose that an investigator has been fortunate enough to find 20 patients fulfilling the requirements for a comparative evaluation of two drugs, D_1 and D_2, respectively. D_1 on the basis of its prior availability has assumed the role of a standard treatment for some particular symptom, while D_2 is a somewhat newer drug, which is claimed by the manufacturer, on the basis of animal experimentation and some preliminary trials with humans, to be superior to D_1 for treatment of the same symptom.

Next, assume that the 20 patients have been divided appropriately into two groups of 10 each, the first assigned to D_1, and the second assigned to D_2. For the main purpose of this example, I shall not consider the question of blinds, or double blinds, or other complications, so that it may be assumed that I am so far dealing with a valid design. For the same purpose, I assume a symptom which is either there or not, and one whose presence or absence is easy to determine. Further, it is assumed that all 20 of the patients have the symptom just prior to the start of treatment, and that none has been under treatment for the symptom before—that is, has had no contact with D_1 or D_2. What I have set up thus far is an almost ideal situation strictly from a design point of view, with one very important exception—the limitation on the number of patients in the study. But, as was noted above, this is a fairly typical kind of limitation in clinical research; and it is surely worth looking at some of the statistical inferential processes which are specifically pertinent to this limitation, and perhaps also at the way in which such processes have been abused beyond logical endurance.

For this purpose I shall assume the following result of this hypothetical drug study: Four out of the 10 patients on D_1 improved, as manifested by the loss of the symptom, compared with 8 of the 10 on D_2.

This ratio of two to one in favor of the new drug, D_2, may cause a flurry of excitement and perhaps a thirty-yard dash to the nearest set of statistical tables for the purpose of testing the null hypothesis that there is no essential difference in effect between the two drugs. The investigator may fervently hope that the tables will show the data to contradict this null hypothesis, thereby establishing a new and better treatment for the symptom, and at the same time making him the proud possessor of a statistically significant result. But all one can do is to utter a sympathetic "Alas." The table will show a significance level of about .17, which seems light-years away from the much coveted .05 level.

More serious than the investigator's personal disappointment at not establishing a statistically significant result is the error in reasoning and in purpose which often accompany the result obtained. The essential usefulness of testing for statistical significance is that it provides a relatively objective procedure for determining whether a particular result, such as the difference between two percentages, *could* have been due to chance alone. However, the failure to obtain a statistically significant result per se does not, even approximately, establish that the difference was in fact due to chance. Yet statements and attitudes verbalized and published day in and day out seem either explicitly or implicitly to convey such an erroneous impression. The seriousness of this distorted interpretation of significance testing can hardly be underestimated. One cannot help but wonder how many valuable leads may have been lost to the argument that what seemed better may after all have just been due to chance.[1]

[1] In the procedure for the testing of hypotheses, statisticians generally recognize two kinds of possible error. In the Type I error the null hypothesis is rejected on the basis of a statistical result when the hypothesis is, in fact, true. The probability with which this kind of error occurs when the null hypothesis is true is directly determined by the chosen level of significance. While the Type I error appears to be generally well understood among clinical investigators who use significance tests, there does appear to be a lack of appreciation for the existence of the Type II error. In the latter, the null hypothesis is accepted as true on the basis of a statistical result, when, in fact, it is false, some alternative hypothesis being true. One of the essential ad-

One of the genuine advantages of significance testing is that it does involve objective mathematical procedures concerning inferences about hypotheses. Perhaps because of the objectivity of the procedures themselves, it is sometimes easy to overlook the degree to which the selection of a hypothesis for testing may be a matter of judgment or—which amounts to the same thing—the fact that it is possible to test any number of hypotheses with the same set of data. To consider an extreme from the same example of 4 out of 10 successes for D_1 against 8 out of 10 for D_2, it would have been possible a priori to test the hypothesis that the true difference between D_2 and D_1 in the percentage of success is .4 in favor of D_2. It is obvious from the data that this hypothesis could not have been refuted, as the result would be entirely nonsignificant. One can then say that the hypothesis concerning the superiority of D_2 over D_1 cannot possibly be rejected on the basis of the particular results. Again, this is not the same as a statement to the effect that the hypothesis of the superiority of D_2 over D_1 is in fact established. In summary, the data in the example, of themselves, can be said to result in the rejection of neither the null hypothesis of equality between the two drugs nor the contradictory null hypothesis asserting the superiority of D_2 over D_1. Yet how often, on the basis of a misinterpretation of the logic of significance testing, does such a set of data result in the rejection of the second of these hypotheses as though it were proved false?

This point is, in theory, just as valid in large sample applications as in designs involving a small number of observations. From a practical point of view, however, in dealing with small samples it seems of much greater importance to understand the logic of significance testing to the extent of avoiding the kind of misinterpretation discussed above. For with a really large sample the failure to obtain a statistically significant difference often can be interpreted to mean that the difference is of no practical significance, either. In fact, even a statistically significant difference obtained from large samples is on occasion seen to be of no practical significance, for the reason that with a sufficiently

---

vantages of a large sample over a small one is that for a fixed Type I error (or level of significance) the probabilities associated with Type II errors are smaller in the larger sample.

large sample even very small differences can be statistically significant.

This is generally not the case in differences obtained from small samples. In the hypothetical example selected above, although the two-to-one ratio of successes of D_2 over D_1 was not statistically significant, such a ratio would be of considerable practical importance if it were representative—that is, if it were maintained in the long run. But I am considering the typical clinical situation in which it is not possible to increase the sample size in conformity with the maintenance of a given design protocol to see whether this ratio will obtain both statistical and "practical" significance.

It should be clear by now that significance tests applied to small samples have, in general, a limited use. If despite the small sample a statistically significant difference is obtained, all well and good. If it is not obtained, but at the same time a difference is obtained which would be both practical and significant had the sample been larger, the significance test applied to such data from a *practical* point of view must be interpreted as rather inconclusive. For a difference which looks impressive, the significance test may show that it could have been due to chance. It does not then say that it *was* due to chance, or even that it was *probably* due to chance.

What does this mean with respect to the application of statistical methodology to clinical design? In trying to answer this question it will be useful to consider the purpose of clinical research on the ward. This is rather a broad subject, but it is worth thinking about in general terms before taking up a more specific example or two. First, such investigation is distinguished by the fact that, as compared with more basic areas of research, it is most directly and immediately related to questions concerning improvement in the treatment of patients. It seems correct to assume that the purpose of all or almost all clinical research on a ward is to obtain results that can be used in some fairly direct way for the treatment of patients on the ward. In planning any such research project, the investigator must ask himself the question, "In what *possible* ways are the results of this study to be used in the subsequent treatment of patients?" At the conclusion of the study he should be able to answer the question,

"In what *specific* ways can I interpret and apply the results of this study to the treatment of patients?"

There is an important difference in spirit between these questions and the more generally conventional ones asked, first, at the outset of a study: "Which null hypotheses do I test?," and at the conclusion, "Which do I reject and, by implication, which do I accept on the basis of the results?" The advantage of the former set of questions is their emphasis on the choice of actions and decisions regarding the actual treatment of patients, in relation to a piece of research. In contrast, the operational aspects of the questions framed in the context of the testing of hypotheses are at best a step removed. One may argue, if one wishes, that the two sets of questions can be regarded as equivalent. But this argument becomes entirely academic, if not facetious, after one draws a random sample from the almost infinite number of hypotheses tested in the recent literature, which provide hardly more than the vaguest hint of what to do.

To return for a few moments to the hypothetical example of D_1 versus D_2, I shall assume that the purpose of the project is not merely to test the null hypothesis that there is no true difference between the old drug D_1 and the new drug D_2, but that a decision is to be made, on the basis of the study, as to whether D_2 should replace D_1 in the subsequent treatment of patients for the symptom in question. To simplify things it may be assumed that no other comparable data exist, and that no other considerations are involved, such as cost, risk of side reaction, and so on. Given this set of conditions and the result of twice as many successes for D_2 as for D_1, it would appear clearly indicated that D_2 is to be preferred, even though there is nonsignificance at the .05 level. That is, in order to have a basis for decision, one requires in such a case an estimate of the true difference in effect between the drugs or of the direction of the difference, whatever the limitation of the sample size.

In statistical terms this means, within the framework of this discussion, that the investigator ought to be concerned with the estimation of parameters rather than, or at least as well as, with the testing of hypotheses. The decision to use D_2 over D_1 does not imply that he has no use at all for the significance test. It is still there to remind him that he could be wrong in his decision to use D_2, even though the use of D_2 is indicated on the basis of the results obtained in the study.

The functional or decision view of clinical design is of considerable importance in questions such as those concerning the use of placeboes. Under what conditions should one use a placebo group of patients within a clinical design? The answer to this question is, of course, not always cut and dried. But even when the answer should be obvious in terms of the limitations on the possible uses of the results of a study, the investigator may be more influenced by some highly idealized conception of what constitutes a good design than by a careful consideration of the use to which the results may be applied.

Consider, for example, a situation in which chlorpromazine is used on a fairly large scale for the treatment of a class of patients in a large mental hospital. A new competing drug is developed by a reputable manufacturer who is eager to test it in a large clinical setting. After some preliminary overtures, the manufacturer's research representative may meet with the responsible clinical investigator of the hospital to discuss the question of clinical design. After they have estimated the number and description of patients who can be made available for the study, questions come up concerning how the patients should be grouped to provide valid comparisons between experimental and control groups, groups on placeboes, and so forth. A popular misconception often appears on the scene at this point, to the effect that such a design should always include a group of patients on placebo. First, it is obvious that, barring some very exceptional or dramatic occurrences, a division of the patients into two groups, one on the new active drug and one on an inactive placebo, will not yield any information for purposes of a valid comparison of the new drug with chlorpromazine. If the purpose of the study is to decide between the new and the old drugs, this kind of design certainly does not suit the purpose.

On the other hand, if one is more interested in obtaining a statistically significant difference at the .05 level per se, the design will be more likely to produce such a result than, say, the operationally more meaningful one in which the patients are divided equally between the new and old drugs, with none on placebo. There are two contributing factors here. First, one would ordinarily expect that the chances for a greater difference in effect would be smaller between two active drugs than between one of them and a placebo. And, second, for a given numerical difference, the significance level would be doubled in the case of the placebo versus the active drug, as opposed to the case of the two active drugs, for the reason that in the former case a one-tailed test is easily justified.

With the realization that for the assumed purpose the design should allow for a valid comparison between the two active drugs, a compromise may be offered, such as a three-way split between chlorpromazine, the new drug, and a placebo, for the feeling may persist that at least some patients should be on a placebo or things aren't really right. The trouble with this is, of course, that it will provide less data for comparing the two active drugs against each other; and even though significance at the .05 level is not the only basis for decision, it is worth trying to achieve such significance within a meaningful framework to the extent that this may be possible. Of course, it has been tacitly assumed that the issue is *not* whether to abandon the use of the drugs altogether. If that were still an open question, or if the data system of the design were developed in a way so as to provide specific comparisons between placebo and nonplacebo groups which could logically and operationally have a bearing on subsequent treatment, then a three-way split to include a placebo group certainly could not be ruled out a priori. (An incidental though perhaps obvious advantage of using one phenothiazine against another rather than against a placebo in double blind studies is perhaps worth mentioning: Such a procedure reduces the chance that the incidence of side reactions will disclose which group of patients is on which treatment.)

I have discussed above a serious limitation of the use of the .05 level of significance as a sole basis for decision when dealing with necessarily small samples, and the kind of logical fallacy which often accompanies the interpretation of a result which is not statistically significant. A second point, which should at least be mentioned, is the application of standard statistical tests of significance applied within the framework of clinical designs where a number of patients in the study are located on the same ward. For this purpose, consider a study confined to a single ward in which patients are randomized into two groups, one on an active drug and the other on a placebo. I shall further assume that the investigator is trying, among other things, to estimate the effect of the drug on a variable which has a recognized aspect of contagion or communicability. That is, here is a situation in which the improvement shown by one patient may per se increase the probability of improvement of a second patient. Returning to the clinical design, I shall assume that the investigator has obtained a difference between the active treatment group and the group on placebo. It can be demonstrated on the basis of some rather elementary mathematical statistical theory that, under the conditions which have been assumed, standard statistical tests based on the assumed statistical independence of the observations—that is, the tests which are used routinely in studies of this kind—*invariably* must understate levels of significance.

This adds insult to injury. For not only is it relatively unlikely that a real difference in effect will achieve statistical significance in a small sample, but one does not even get, by standard tests (and here I include both parametric and nonparametric tests) full credit for the level of significance actually achieved. It is small wonder, then, that so many clinical studies performed on relatively carefully matched groups of patients fail rather miserably when put to the .05 test. These results are then interpreted as being apparently in conflict with everyday clinical experience in the use of one drug or another. It is clear that such alleged conflicts may to a considerable extent be due to the limitations and misinterpretations of current clinical statistical research procedures and methodology, rather than being entirely the fault of the practising nonresearch clinician with his perhaps more obvious biases.

If the only remedy one had was to push forward regardless of the failure to meet .05 levels of significance, then the outlook for progress would, it must be acknowledged, still be rather uncertain, although a clearer awareness of some of the pitfalls of current methodology could not help but be a somewhat liberating phenomenon. Fortunately there is another basic approach to the study of psychopathology—*the intensive statistical study of the individual patient.* This approach can be regarded either as complementary to the one in which degrees of freedom for statistical inferences depend entirely on the number of patients in a study, or as basic on its own merits.

It is hard to understand why the intensive individual approach has been so completely neglected in formal clinical research. One must conclude that the reason for this failure probably results from a general misunderstanding, or at best a haziness, about the inferential possibilities of the much maligned "individual case." It is certainly not as generally recognized as it ought to be that *the intensive statistical study of a single case can provide more meaningful and statistically significant information than, say, only end-point observations extended over a relatively large number of patients.*

I should like to consider again two groups of 10 patients each, the first on an active drug and the second on a placebo. An earlier example showed that, even if there were twice as many successes on the drug as on the placebo, the .05 level of significance would still not be reached. While the investigator may still go ahead and use the drug, for practical purposes considering it to have a real effect, he should not be too surprised if later experience produces evidence that the experimental result not only could have been due to chance, but apparently was. Thus the results from the experimental design at its conclusion lack statistical proof that the drug was really effective. In concrete terms, this means that, although the evidence does favor the drug and it might be used on that basis, the investigator is not certain that it was actually helpful at all to even a single one of the 10 patients who were on it. It is necessary to appreciate fully the importance of this conclusion, which results from a statistically nonsignificant difference based on end-point observations with degrees of freedom based only on the number of patients.

Now I should like to consider in brief outline an intensive statistical study of a single patient with respect to the use of the drug. To implement such a design, I shall assume that I am dealing with a variable or a symptom which has a degree of variability within the individual patient over time. This is not an unreasonable assumption, since many of the important behavioral and psychopathological traits have this property—which, incidentally, to some extent may be regarded as contributing to the over-all problem of reliability. I shall discuss this more fully later.

If one observes the patient over sufficiently long periods, with placebo and without placebo, varying the treatment either randomly or systematically, depending on various relevant considerations, one can, in general, over a sufficient period of time obtain a sufficiently large number of observations to achieve statistical significance, if, in fact, a true difference does exist; and also to obtain an accurate measure of this difference—that is, to obtain relatively precise estimates of parameters. I shall assume that an investigator has performed such an experimental design and that the results were statistically significant. *He then has shown, with but a single case, that the drug has had a real effect —a positive statement which could not be made in the previous instance, with 20 cases and a ratio of two to one. Moreover, not only has a genuine effect been demonstrated, but along with this some rather specific parameters and accompanying background factors have been delineated.* Since the patient's age, his specific symptomatology, various of his measurable physiological characteristics, and so on, are known, the investigator has learned something definite about the particular values of these variables, in whose presence the significant result was possible. He has at the very least learned that none of these specific values and characteristics was per se capable of negating the definite significant result that was obtained.

Now it might be argued that all the investigator knows is that the drug has had a statistically significant effect on a single patient; there is no proof that the drug will be a help beyond that case. While this assertion is logically true, it should be recalled, first, that the investigator has established statistically that the effect of the drug on the single case was not due to chance. Therefore, it is not unreasonable to assume that there exist other patients, in particular those with one or another characteristic, or a combination of characteristics, similar to the case in the design, who would also respond significantly to the same treatment. *From the point of view of statistical inference per se the intensive single case study can be considered as providing data sampled from a statistical distribution or population defined by the set of particular parameters or characteristics of the patient under study.* One has no a priori knowledge that the same kind of result will appear in a second patient with the same relevant or presumably relevant characteristics; one's expectation of a similarity of result depends simply on the assumption that this second patient is representative of a population or statistical distribution sufficiently close to that of the design patient to permit inferences from the one to the other.

This ability to specify background and other characteristics in relation to the results of a study is almost completely lost when one relies on extensive rather than intensive designs. The parameters and characteristics of the extensive study are necessarily vague. The heterogeneity of characteristics in even minimal extensive samples inevitably results in a corresponding vagueness concerning the specification of the population characteristics and background variables about which inferences can be made. At best, there can be only a rough averaging in the midst of generally unavoidable and hidden statistical biases. This is obviously in marked contrast to the intensive statistical study of the individual case. *Thus the argument cited against generalization to other patients, from the result of a single case intensively studied, can actually be applied in a more realistic and devastating manner against the value of inferences which are customarily drawn from studies in which extensive rather than intensive degrees of freedom are used*—that is, where *n* is based on the number of patients rather than on the number of observations of a single patient. This is particularly true when one seeks to apply the results of a study to a treatment program.

I should now like to assume that the investigator has been able to get a fairly large extensive sample, and a difference in effect which was statistically significant at the .05 level. What are the nature and limitations of the inferences which can then be drawn? First, if he wishes to draw inferences from the results of such a study to a class or population of patients in a way which utilizes the large number of patients, he is hard pressed to establish a reasonably homogeneous or operationally useful population for such inferences. If he is lucky enough to get as many as 50 patients for his study, he may be able to describe his sample as consisting of "50 chronic schizophrenic patients, aged 31–60; period of hospitalization, 2–12 years," and so on. These are rather wide variations, but quite typical for these and other possibly relevant variables among a group of 50 patients selected for a study. Any one or more of such variables may a priori have an important influence on the success of treatment.

With this in mind I should like to return to the assumed fact of the statistical significance of the results. In the first place, it is obvious that if one were to enumerate the particular patients who apparently improved on the drug, such improvement with respect to the individual patient could not be interpreted as significant in the same sense as in a study based on an intensive individual design. *That is, in the extensive model, regardless of the significance level, the particular patients who were on the drug and who benefited from the drug cannot be distinguished from the patients who were on the drug but who benefited by chance.* Significance here is necessarily in terms of an average over a wide range of individuals and their parameters, and the greater the heterogeneity of the design sample, the less the data indicate for which values of the parameters in the samples the effect was real.

For example, suppose that the investigator was even fortunate enough to be able to balance his drug and his placebo group for age, and that he had 5 patients in each group between the ages of 50 and 60. Now it is quite unlikely, except with a rather dramatic difference in results with respect to this age group within this study, that he would obtain an answer to as simple and yet operationally important a question as, "Is the active treatment of any possible value in the specific treatment of a patient in the age group of 50 to 60?" The same limitation will, in general, be true of other relevant variables, given the usual degree of heterogeneity in a sample of that size. On the other hand, a statistically significant result in the single-case intensive design specifies a set of patient-variables according to the description of the patient which accompanied the significant change, and which therefore delineates more distinctly the particular values of the parameters which accompanied successful treatment.

A further obvious limitation of the extensive model is that all of the possibly important patient variables are unlikely to be balanced between the experimental and the control group. Some rather serious imbalances, either hidden or manifest, may easily occur, so that the significance level itself can be spurious. This kind of bias can, of course, work either way—against significance or in its favor. Such biases are obviously minimized, if not actually eliminated, in the intensive model, where a patient can serve as his own control.

A very important aspect of the intensive approach is that in the process of increasing the number of patients studied intensively for such obvious purposes as verification, validation, modification, and extension of results, *the clinical investigator has a far greater opportunity to achieve a sense of direction and a steady progress than he could possibly have in a succession of extensive studies. He can select patients in a systematic way with respect to various characteristics and background factors, and can move more steadily in the direction of increasingly precise statements than he could ever hope to do on the basis of extensive studies.* The continuing selection of patients for intensive statistical study can in practice and in theory be much more closely related in a meaningful way to previous results. *Intensive studies thus permit a more integrated approach to clinical research on the ward.*

The advantages of an intensive statistical system for the study of the individual patient, and its application to groups of individual patients, extend beyond the particular technical questions of logic and correct statistical inference and the rather direct operational consequences of them which have been discussed explicitly so far. For example, in the field of the ataractics, it is only through frequent observations on each patient over periods of sufficient duration that one can ever hope to secure useful data concerning the distribution of optimal dosage levels in relation to specific patient characteristics and goals. At what point, and with respect to which patient characteristics and symptoms, will an increase in dosage level introduce a risk of a side reaction of one description or another? At what point might an increase move the patient from one extreme of psychopathology to its opposite, and so forth?

In a fairly recent and rather large-scale extensive study, in which an attempt was presumably made to test one ataractic against another, the dosage level throughout the course of the study was held constant. An immediate limitation here is that, regardless of what data system is to be used in such a study, whatever comparisons are to be made between the drugs can obviously be valid only with respect to the fixed dosage level. Furthermore, the dosage level selected was one that the investigators decided would be sufficiently low to reduce, if not eliminate, the probability of a side reaction which might cause a drop-out from the study, thus making the statistical analysis of the data even less useful than it would otherwise be. But what about simply ruling out the possible comparison of side effects?

It seems at least possible that the superiority of one ataractic agent over another may lie in the reduction of the risk of a side reaction. Concerning drop-outs, these are perhaps exactly the cases about which one can learn the most concerning counter-indications. *After all, in actual clinical practice, higher dosages will be given, side reactions will occur, and patients will be taken off a drug,* but the rather expensive piece of research to which I have been referring was *carefully designed not to impart any information about these rather crucial phenomena—this, in addition to not providing any data about the possible beneficial effects, if any, on higher dosage levels, such as are actually used in clinical practice.*

The fault is not necessarily a lack of ingenuity of the clinical investigator, but rather one of the severe limitations of the extensive model. In general, intensive individual studies permit a greater elasticity in the use of dosage levels, and are thereby more operationally useful with respect to the applicability of the results. For example, data accumulated with respect to each patient in an intensive design, by virtue of the frequency of observation over time, allow the possibility of securing information relevant to drop-out in a systematic and operationally useful way.

The development of intensive statistical systems and clinical designs based on frequent observations of each patient offers fresh approaches to the treatment of reliability. While I have discussed this in some detail in other papers, the main points may be worth summarizing in the present context.

First, there are two essential types of reliability which have been of concern to clinical research methodologists. The first has been called test-retest reliability, and the second, interobserver reliability. Briefly, the most prevalent point of view about test-retest reliability is that the result of tests or clinical examinations administered to the same patient or group of patients at two successive and relatively close points in time should be in reasonably close agreement, as measured by a coefficient of correlation, or some similar statistic. The absence of such agreement is viewed as a serious limitation of the test, examination, or instrument and may be followed by discard of the instrument and search for a new one. There is a second approach which appears more fruitful, and which may prevent the running-out of time and of instruments. This follows from the consideration that, in general, there is considerable clinical evidence of a basic variability from one period to the next in the manifestation of psychopathological characteristics in the same patient, and that valid operational definitions of the patient-state consequently require, particularly for research purposes, the incorporation of such variability. Thus much of what may appear as a deficiency in a measuring instrument, insofar as test-retest reliability is concerned, may be a reflection of the probabilistic aspect of the patient-state. But even if an instrumental defect is involved, provided the instrument is considered generally valid for the purpose of its use, *the frequency of observation with respect to each patient under study cannot help but increase the over-all precision of the measurement system.*

The question of reliability which is defined in terms of agreement between observers is apparently a more difficult problem. A promising approach to the handling of interobserver reliability is, however, again to be found in the development of intensive data systems for the study of each patient. With respect to a number of possible variables to be studied in one intensive data system or another, one requires a design in which several observers independently report intensively on a single patient, as well as a design in which one observer reports intensively on several patients, individually and over sufficient time periods, and in which the observers themselves are considered as part of the instrumentation, each with his own random error and possible systematic bias.

This kind of design may be looked at in two distinct though related ways. From a conventional point of view, it simply allows one to adjust for individual observer bias and to average observer biases. From another, perhaps Sullivanian, point of view, one may consider each observer-patient pair over time as generating an interpersonal field, and each set of observer-patient pairs, consisting of the same patient but with different observers, as the totality of fields under observation in a study with respect to a given patient. If now one considers in particular a variable of the system, the variability in the rating between observers with respect to a fixed patient may perhaps be more advantageously viewed as a measure of the variability in the interpersonal fields generated by the patient, than as always necessarily being a simple matter of observer bias. One might, for example, conclude that consistent responses from observer to observer and over time with respect to certain of their ratings on a given patient may reflect a stereotypic response pattern of one sort or another by the patient, rather than a particular reliability of the instrument and the observers. By the same argument an apparent lack of agreement either over time *or* between observers may reflect a loss or lack of stereotypic response and accordingly be indicative of a relatively healthy state in the patient rather than of poor reliability in general. On the other hand, depending on the particular variable in question and the rating, it is of course also possible that complete agreement by the observers may reflect the healthier state.

While the validity of the intensive design which was briefly outlined above does not depend upon this particular application of Sullivan's field concepts to experimental design, it nevertheless may be regarded as entirely consistent with it.

The acceptance of the validity of intensive statistical studies of the individual patient, and of groups of patients in the setting of the mental hospital, requires a changing attitude toward the use of data systems which appear to attempt to include every conceivably observable or inferential event with the slightest hint of possible relevance to the study of psychopathology. It is no longer a mark of sophistication to show an appreciation of the apparent high order of dimensionality of events which may have a bearing on one or another aspect of psychopathology. But it is something less than sophisticated to believe that one can, in a given study, benefit by the use of statistical systems in which the number of variables exceed the available degrees of freedom by a factor of one thousand. This appears to be another unfortunate feature of many an extensive model. Besides the technical statistical limitations to the analysis of such hyperdimensionalized and often contrived data systems, there are the more obvious physical and mental limitations, including the consideration that the larger the number of really distinct items an observer has to rate within a given allotted period of observation and reporting, the less likely he is to achieve a generally acceptable level of true reliability—that is, in this case, reliability in the sense of precision of observation. In the application of intensive clinical designs, the use of such hyperdimensionalized data systems must be ruled out a priori, as a matter of practicality as well as correct technical statistical methodology.

Thus far in this presentation, very little has been said concerning statistical techniques pertinent to the analysis of intensive designs. One can, as a first approximation, use the same techniques used in extensive models, but with greater emphasis on estimation rather than merely on the testing of null hypotheses—an improvement which is possible on the basis of the larger *n* available for intensive studies. However, the more dynamic models found in the statistical literature under the headings of stochastic processes and time-series analysis seem more appropriate as models for intensive designs. The Markov chain model is perhaps the simplest and most direct within the context of a nonparametric approach. In recent years a number of technical statistical papers have offered procedures for estimating parameters and testing hypotheses with respect to these models, and some of these procedures provide an excellent technical point of origin for intensive clinical designs.

To sum up some of my main points, the validity and general usefulness of what seems to be a common practice in formal experimental designs in ward settings is open to serious question. This is the practice of testing hypotheses between groups of patients in which the total number of degrees of freedom cannot exceed the number of patients in the study. A severe limitation of such extensive models lies, first, in the necessarily relatively small number of patients which practical considerations and other limiting factors often impose. Under such limitations, it is often quite difficult to obtain a statistically significant difference, although the difference actually obtained may be quite large.

The failure to reject the null hypothesis is often mistaken by the research investigator as logically or statistically equivalent to establishing it. Lack of appreciation of this perhaps subtle distinction must lie behind many a statement by the research investigator that some active drug was no better than a placebo, when such a statement conflicts with the everyday experience of the clinician. *It is quite possible that biases resulting from the misinterpretation of statistical inferential procedures on the part of the methodologists of clinical design have contributed as much as, if not more than, the individual biases of the clinician to the general confusion about the effect of tranquilizers.* While most investigators are alert to the possibility of error due to individual clinical bias, there is much less of an awareness of errors in inference. A critical examination of the literature will show that such errors in inference—or in the assumed operational implication of the results—are quite common in applications of the extensive design.

Further errors in inference may occur with regard to the extensive model in the statement of significance levels themselves, because of lack of statistical independence of the observations. For example, when standard statistical procedures are used, the significance level of the difference between two means will always be understated with respect to a given observed difference, if the tested variable is one which is contagious or communicable, as is actually the case with many of the important variables in the study of behavior and affect. This is a factor which strengthens the methodological bias against the detection or utilization of true effects.

Even with the achievement of statistical significance in the extensive model, there are severe limitations in terms of identifying many of the possibly relevant patient characteristics and parameters associated with the statistically significant result. This is a product of the vagueness of the population which the patients in the design are supposed to represent as a sample. This lack of specificity is the result of the heterogeneity of the data, which, in general, tends to increase with increases in the number of patients needed to establish a given difference as significant.

It is, moreover, quite difficult to obtain strictly comparable groups of patients for use in an extensive model. Manifest or hidden differences in patient characteristics, in view of the necessarily small sample sizes, can play havoc with significance levels in either direction—in favor of or against significance. This is in marked contrast to intensive designs, where patients can be used as their own controls.

On the other hand, *the use of intensive models which are based on frequent observations of the individual patient over periods of sufficiently long duration is a basic methodological approach which can overcome the essential limitations of the extensive model.* It permits the valid testing of hypotheses and the estimation of parameters with far greater precision and flexibility. The population of reference from the intensive data of a single case is well specified, and the influence of various patient characteristics on the outcome of treatment can be studied with a directness which cannot possibly be achieved in the extensive model. Consequently, judgments concerning indications for treatment, as well as for continuing research involving the use of such data, are far more operationally meaningful than is the case in the extensive model, and the results of intensive studies can have more direct and immediate implications for improvement in the treatment of patients than is generally possible from the result of extensive studies. This quality of the intensive model further allows for a greater sense of direction and a superior approach to a well-integrated program of clinical research than is otherwise possible.

3

Statistics for the Investigation of Individual Cases* †

R. W. PAYNE and H. GWYNNE JONES

PROBLEM

Much of the work of a clinical psychologist consists of making relatively routine psychological measurements of fairly well established traits, either cognitive or orectic. It is well known, however, that there can be no measurement without error. The psychologist must have the means of taking error into account if he is to assess his test scores intelligently. There appear to be three main types of question which face clinical psychologists:

1. The Abnormality of a Discrepancy between Two Scores

This problem arises every time a psychologist gives more than one measure. Perhaps the commonest example is the Wechsler-Bellevue Intelligence Scale. This test provides two rather different measures of intelligence, the "Verbal Scale IQ" and the "Performance Scale IQ." It is a common experience that these two scores are divergent. In fact the discrepancy may suggest interesting hypotheses in line with other abnormalities the patient shows. However, before we can assess such a discrepancy, we must taken into account two factors. We know that neither scale

---

* Reprinted from the *Journal of Clinical Psychology,* 1957, Vol. 13, No. 2, pp. 115–121, by permission of the authors and the publisher.

† Editorial Note: The authors use the term "standard error of prediction" which is customarily called a "standard error estimate" in America, and in this country we uniformly refer to the "proportions" or "probabilities" corresponding to various standard score values instead of the term "percentile."

is perfectly reliable and we also know that the scales are not perfectly correlated. Therefore, many normal people would show discrepancies between the two scales which one need not take seriously. The first question we can ask ourselves then, is how frequently would a discrepancy as large as the one we observe occur in the normal population? That is, how "abnormal" is the difference we observe between our test scores?

2. *The Reliability of a Discrepancy between Two Scores*

In certain cases, we may have occasion to give two tests which measure rather different traits. For example, we may give a test of long term retention, and a test of general intelligence. It may be the case that these tests have a very low intercorrelation in the general population, so that quite large discrepancies between these scores could be quite "normal" or usual in the general population. Nevertheless, on clinical grounds, we might expect our patient to have a lower memory test score than a general intelligence test score. We are not implying that this would be an abnormally *large* discrepancy. Many people may have as large differences. We *are* implying, however, that it is a *measurable* difference. We know that neither test is perfectly reliable, so that small differences will occur by "chance." What we wish to know is how large a difference between any two scores must be before we can be sure the difference could not be due merely to error of measurement of the tests.

3. *Testing a Clinical Prediction*

A third type of problem is slightly different. Very often the clinical psychologist finds himself repeating a measurement with a certain expectation or "prediction." For example, a patient may obtain an "average" IQ when first seen. Two years later, there may be strong clinical grounds for believing that deterioration has taken place. We, therefore, wish to retest him on the same (or a similar) test of intelligence to confirm the hypothesis that he has deteriorated. We may, indeed, find that his score is now below average. Have we in fact confirmed our hypothesis?

Again we know that tests are not perfectly reliable and that such changes in score occur in perfectly normal people. Essentially we need a control group. We need to know what proportion of individuals like our patient, of the same IQ on the first test, and who have *not* deteriorated would show an equal drop in IQ on retest. If the figure is fairly large, of course, our result does not prove that deterioration has really occurred. The practising psychologist will not have time to conduct the appropriate control experiment. Is there any other way of providing an approximate answer?

SUGGESTED SOLUTIONS

The clinical teaching section of the Institute of Psychiatry (Maudsley Hospital) became aware of these problems several years ago. The following simple statistical models were eventually evolved and have since been applied routinely in clinical practice.

1. The Abnormality of a Discrepancy between Two Scores

Let us call the two raw scores X and Y. We are required to discover how frequently a discrepancy or difference between them occurs in the general population. Let us call this difference D, which is merely $X - Y$. Provided that the bi-variate distribution of the two scores is normal, the percentile value for any D score can be obtained from the ordinary table of the normal curve relating percentiles to standard scores. All we need to do, is to express our D score as a standard score in the usual way, substituting in the formula:

$$Z_d \text{ (standard ``}D\text{'' score)} = \frac{D - \overline{D}}{\sigma_d}$$

In this equation $D = X - Y$, $\overline{D}$ (mean D) $= \overline{X} - \overline{Y}$, and σ_d (standard error of difference, or standard deviation of the D scores) =

$$\sqrt{\sigma_x^2 + \sigma_y^2 - 2r_{xy}\sigma_x\sigma_y}$$

Where σ_x is of course the standard deviation of test x, σ_y the standard deviation of test y, and r_{xy} the Pearson product-moment correlation between tests x and y.

This general method will tell us how frequently this particular D score occurs in the standardization population. Our D score, however, was the difference between two raw scores, and as such is influenced by both X and Y. If, however, test x has a very much larger standard deviation (and range) than test y, score D will be influenced much more by score X than score Y (*i.e.*, D scores will correlate higher with X than with Y scores). In an extreme case, an "abnormally" (infrequently) large X score would automatically produce an "abnormally" large D score. This would be the case if raw X and Y scores are used. Psychologically, however, we are not really concerned with the discrepancy between raw X and Y scores, as raw scores on most psychological tests are quite arbitrary. What we are concerned with is a discrepancy between the *percentile* standing on test x and the *percentile* standing on test y. Thus, it is really the "abnormality" (frequency) of a discrepancy between two percentiles that concerns us. We can easily estimate this if we first express our raw X and Y scores as *standard* scores, and then assess the frequency of the difference between these two standard scores in the general population.

Thus, we can first transform our raw X and Y scores into standard scores according to the formulae:

$$Z_x = \frac{X - \overline{X}}{\sigma_x} \quad \text{and} \quad Z_y = \frac{Y - \overline{Y}}{\sigma_y}$$

We can then find the difference between the two standard scores: $D_z = Z_x - Z_y$ (D_z = difference between standard scores). This difference (discrepancy) can then itself be expressed as a standard score, so that its percentile position can be ascertained:

$$Z_{d_z} = \frac{D_z - \overline{D}_z}{\sqrt{\sigma_{z_x}{}^2 + \sigma_{z_y}{}^2 - 2r_{xy}\sigma_{z_x}\sigma_{z_y}}}$$

However, $\overline{D}_z$ (the *mean* difference between standard scores of x and y) is zero, as standard scores are made to have a mean of zero. Similarly σ_{z_x} (the standard deviation of Z_x or x standard scores), is one, as standard scores are made to have a standard deviation of one. Thus:

$$Z_{d_z} = \frac{Z_x - Z_y}{\sqrt{1 + 1 - 2r_{xy}}}$$

By consulting the tables for the normal curve, we can transform this Z into a percentile and discover how frequently the difference occurs in the general population. A "two tailed" test tells us how frequently a discrepancy of this magnitude or greater between the two standard scores occurs in the general population, regardless of the direction of the discrepancy. A "one tailed" test tells us how frequently the difference occurs in this particular direction (for example how frequently Z_x exceeds Z_y by this degree in the population).

Example. A man of 25 obtains a Wechsler (*6*) Verbal Scale IQ of 120, and a Wechsler Performance Scale IQ of 105. We wish to know how common such a large discrepancy actually is. We know that the mean of both Wechsler scales is 100, and the standard deviation is 15. Thus, the Verbal Score, expressed as a standard score $= \frac{120 - 100}{15} = 1.33$. The Performance IQ expressed as a standard score is $\frac{105 - 100}{15} = 0.33$.

The difference between these two standard scores (Verbal minus Performance) is 1.00. The correlation between the Wechsler Verbal IQ and Performance Scale IQ is 0.71 (*6*, p. 124).[1] Thus the standard error of the difference between these two Wechsler standard scores would be:

$$\sqrt{1 + 1 - 2(0.71)} = 0.762$$

Dividing the difference (minus the mean difference—in this case zero) by the standard error of the difference, we find that:

$$Z = \frac{1.00}{0.762} = 1.31$$

Consulting the table for converting standard scores into percentiles (*2*, p. 359) we see that this corresponds to a percentile

[1] We would not use the volue of .83 which Wechsler also quotes after correction for attenuation, as we are concerned here with the empirically found range of verbal-performance discrepancies in the standardization population.

value of 90.5. Thus we see that 19% of the standardization population would have a discrepancy this large (or larger) between Verbal and Performance IQ (the "two tailed" test); 9.5% of the standardization population would have a discrepancy this large (or larger) in favor of the Verbal IQ, as in this case; and 9.5% of the standardization population would have a discrepancy this large (or larger) in favor of the Performance IQ (the "one tailed" test). Whether this discrepancy is infrequent enough in the general population to be regarded as "abnormal," and perhaps worthy of further investigation, must be left to the judgment of the individual clinical psychologist.

2. *The Reliability of a Discrepancy between Two Scores*

Let us again call the two raw scores X and Y. We are required to discover whether the discrepancy between them (D, or $X - Y$) is large enough to be outside the range of differences attributable to the errors of measurement of the two tests. The "standard error of measurement" is the usual psychological estimate of the range of error which we can expect from a single test. The standard error of measurement is usually defined according to the formula:

$$\text{S.E.}_{\cdot m} = \sigma_x\sqrt{1 - r_{xx}}$$

where r_{xx} refers to the coefficient of reliability of the test concerned. This is either a test-retest product moment correlation coefficient, a "split-half" product moment correlation coefficient corrected for attenuation, or sometimes a form *vs.* form correlation coefficient.

If we accept the equation for the standard error of measurement, then the probability of an obtained score "X" on any test departing from a given score which we could call "T" through error of measurement, can easily be obtained according to the formula:

$$Z = \frac{X - T}{\sigma_x\sqrt{1 - r_{xx}}}$$

Thus $(\sigma_x\sqrt{1 - r_{xx}})^2$ represents the error variance of test x.

However, we know that the standard error of a *difference* between two scores X and Y is given by the formula:

$$\text{S.E. diff} = \sqrt{\sigma_x^2 + \sigma_y^2 - 2r\sigma_x\sigma_y}$$

If we replace the variance of X by the error variance of X and the variance of Y by the error variance of Y in the above equation, we will estimate the standard error of the differences attributable solely to error. As error is uncorrelated, however, the last term $(-2r\sigma_x\sigma_y)$ will become zero. (Errors of measurement on test x are uncorrelated with errors on test y). Thus the standard deviation of the discrepancies between X and Y attributable solely to *error of measurement* as defined, will be given by the formula:

$$\sigma \text{ error diff} = \sqrt{(\sigma_x\sqrt{1 - r_{xx}})^2 + (\sigma_y\sqrt{1 - r_{yy}})^2}$$

If we wish to determine the probability of any difference $(X - Y)$ between two scores being due solely to the errors of measurement of the two tests, we can thus set up the following ratio:

$$Z = \frac{D - \bar{D}}{\sqrt{(\sigma_x\sqrt{1 - r_{xx}})^2 + (\sigma_y\sqrt{1 - r_{yy}})^2}}$$

where:

$$D = X - Y \quad \text{and} \quad \bar{D} = \bar{X} - \bar{Y}$$

As we have seen, however, D, the difference between X and Y in raw scores, can be correlated much more highly with X than with Y, if σ_x is much greater than σ_y. In an extreme case for example, where the range of X is very much larger than the range of Y, an extremely high X score would always be "reliably" different from a Y score of *any* value, whatever the reliability of test Y, if the above formula were used. In other words, the judgment of whether or not the difference D were large enough to be measurable, would be almost entirely a function of the size of X. This is clearly not what is required. Again, this difficulty can be surmounted if we first equalize the variance of X and Y by converting both scores to standard scores. We can then apply the formula above, and obtain a valid answer. In standard score units, the formula becomes:

$$Z = \frac{D_z - \bar{D}_z}{\sqrt{(\sqrt{1 - r_{xx}})^2 + (\sqrt{1 - r_{yy}})^2}}$$

$$= \frac{D_z}{\sqrt{(1 - r_{xx}) + (1 - r_{yy})}}$$

where:

$$D_z = Z_x - Z_y,\ \bar{D}_z = \bar{Z}_x - \bar{Z}_y = 0,$$

r_{xx} = coefficient of reliability of test x, and

r_{yy} = coefficient of reliability of test y.

Our standard score, Z, can be converted into a percentile by consulting the table for the normal curve in the usual way.

Example. A male patient of 20 was given the "General Aptitude Test Battery" of the United States Employment Service (5). It was expected from his Wechsler results that his Spatial Aptitude would be higher than his "G" score on the GATB. He obtained a "G" score of 75 and a "Spatial" score of 86. We wish to discover whether or not this difference is in fact measurable, that is, whether a difference this large is within the range of differences one might expect from error of measurement.

If we call the "Spatial" score "X" and the "G" score "Y", we can first convert these scores into standard scores. We know that for both these tests, the mean is 100 and the standard deviation is 20. Thus:

$$Z_x = \frac{X - \bar{X}}{\sigma_x} = \frac{86 - 100}{20} = -0.70$$

and

$$Z_y = \frac{Y - \bar{Y}}{\sigma_y} = \frac{75 - 100}{20} = -1.25$$

The coefficient of reliability of the Spatial test (test "X") is .88, and the coefficient of the "G" test (test "Y") is .94. These are test-retest reliability coefficients quoted in the test manual (5, pp. 1–4) for a male population comparable to the patient. We can now substitute in the equation:

$$Z = \frac{D_z}{\sqrt{(1 - r_{xx}) + (1 - r_{yy})}} \quad \text{where } D_z = Z_x - Z_y$$

$$= \frac{0.55}{\sqrt{(1 - 0.88) + (1 - 0.94)}} = \frac{0.55}{0.424} = 1.30$$

Consulting the table for the normal curve we find that a Z of 1.30 corresponds to a percentile value of 90.3. Thus differences as large or larger than our eleven point discrepancy between "G" and "Spatial" scores could occur 19.4% of the time through error of measurement alone. Differences in the expected direction (*i.e.*, "Spatial" higher than "G") could occur 9.7% of the time through error of measurement (the one tail test). Thus we cannot be certain that this test discrepancy represents a "real" difference between these two aptitudes, and the assessment of these probabilities must again be left to the individual clinician.

3. *Testing a Clinical Prediction*

If we have given a certain test to a patient, and expect a drop in score following some trauma or other circumstance, and subsequently retest our patient on the same test, we wish to discover what proportion of subjects, all of whom had the same initial score on the test, but who did *not* suffer the trauma, would be expected to show a drop this large. This is a relatively simple matter, if we have the relevant data for the test in question. What is required is the test-retest data for the test over an equivalent period of time, for a representative sample of subjects similar to the patient. In other words, our patient's original test score must fall within the distribution of scores obtained by our statistical "control group" on the initial testing.

Let us call the initial test score X, and the score obtained on retest, Y. The regression line of Y upon X is that straight line which best fits (by "least squares") the points represented by the *mean* Y score of each group (column) of subjects with homogeneous X scores. If we use $\hat{Y}$ to represent that Y score which would be predicted from the regression equation from our patient's X (initial test) score, then $\hat{Y}$ also represents the *mean* Y score (retest score) of all those subjects who started out with the same X (initial test) score as our patient. It is this group then, which serves as our patient's "control" group. The *standard error of prediction* using this regression equation represents the standard deviation of the Y (retest) scores of all those patients who started out with the same X (test) score as our patient. We have only to determine then, whether our patient's Y (retest) score falls within or outside the distribution of Y (retest) scores obtained by those people with the same initial X (test score.

In practice then, we would first discover the *average* Y (retest) score of those people with the same initial X (test) score as our patient, by substituting in the regression equation:

$$\hat{Y} = a + bX \quad \text{where } a = \overline{Y} - b\overline{X} \quad \text{and} \quad b = r_{xy}\frac{\sigma_y}{\sigma_x}$$

$\hat{Y}$ = mean retest (Y) score of people who start out with score X
X = patient's initial score
$\overline{X}$ = Mean of all subjects on test X (test)
$\overline{Y}$ = Mean of all subjects on test Y (retest)
σ_x = standard deviation of all subjects on test X (test)
σ_y = standard deviation of all subjects on test Y (retest)
r_{xy} = product moment correlation between test x and test y (*i.e.*, test-retest correlation)

Having discovered our value for $\hat{Y}$, we can then discover the *standard deviation* of the Y scores (retest scores) of those people with the same initial X (test) score. This is the standard error of prediction, and is merely:

$$\text{S.E.}_{\text{predic.}} = \sigma_y\sqrt{1 - r_{xy}^2}$$

Having obtained this value, we merely determine whether our patient's score falls within or outside this group of retest scores for people with the same initial score, by expressing our subject's score as a standard score for this distribution according to the formula:

$$Z = \frac{Y - \hat{Y}}{\text{S.E.}_{\text{predic.}}}$$

The final Z value can be converted to a percentile by consulting the standard table of the normal curve. Since a prediction has been made in each case where this statistical model is used, a *one tailed* test of significance is appropriate.

Example. A 30 year old schizophrenic patient is given the Wechsler Bellevue Form I, and obtains a total weighted score of 110 (IQ = 112). He is believed to have deteriorated intellectually following treatment with Serpasil, and is retested one month later. He now obtains a total weighted score of 83 (IQ = 94) on Wechsler Form I. We wish to discover how many schizophrenics of this initial IQ who have *not* had any treatment intervening between test and retest on the Wechsler over a four week period, would have dropped to this extent.

Some control data is given in an article by Hamister (*1*) who tested a group of 34 schizophrenics on Wechsler I and retested them four weeks later. Their mean total weighted score on the first test was 92.97, with a S.D. of 26.00. Their mean total weighted score on retest was 104.26, with a S.D. of 28.91. The correlation between test and retest was .84.

First we must use the regression equation to discover what the average retest score ($\hat{Y}$ in the formula) was in Hamister's group, for patients with the same initial Wechsler score:

$$\hat{Y} = a + bX \quad \text{where } a = \overline{Y} - b\overline{X} \quad \text{and} \quad b = r_{xy}\frac{\sigma_y}{\sigma_x}$$

We know that $\overline{Y} = 104.26$ (retest mean), $\overline{X} = 92.97$, $\sigma_y = 28.91$, $\sigma_x = 26.00$, $r_{xy} = .84$, and X (patient's initial score) = 110, and Y (patient's retest score) = 83.

Therefore:

$$b = 0.84 \times \frac{28.91}{26.00} = 0.93$$

and:

$$a = 104.26 - (0.93 \times 92.97) = 17.80$$

Thus:

$$\hat{Y} = 17.80 + (0.93 \times 110) = 120.10$$

The standard deviation of retest (Y) scores of schizophrenics with this initial X score is given by the formula:

$$\begin{aligned} \text{S.E.}_{\text{predic.}} &= \sigma_y\sqrt{1 - r_{xy}^2} \\ &= 28.91\sqrt{1 - 84^2} \\ &= 15.69 \end{aligned}$$

Thus the patient's standard score position in the distribution of retest scores obtained by patients with the same initial test score is given by the formula:

$$Z = \frac{Y - \hat{Y}}{\text{S.E.}_{\text{predic.}}}$$

$$= \frac{83 - 120.10}{15.69}$$

$$= -2.37$$

Consulting the table for the normal curve, this is equivalent to a percentile value of 1. Thus we see that only 1% of the schizophrenics in the "control" sample who started out with this IQ on the Wechsler, would have dropped as much on retest after four weeks as has our patient. This is consistent with our hypothesis that he has deteriorated.

SUMMARY

This paper suggests simple statistical models for use in solving the following problems:

1. To estimate how large a discrepancy between any two test scores need be, for it to be "abnormally" large in the standardization population. That is, to estimate the frequency of occurrence in the standardization population of any given discrepancy between two test scores.
2. To establish how large a difference between two test scores need be, for it to be outside the range of differences produced solely by the errors of measurement of the two tests. That is to estimate how large a discrepancy must be for us to judge it a "measurable" difference.
3. To estimate how large a predicted change in score (following treatment, trauma, etc.) need be, to lie outside the range of changes found in a control group which has not been subjected to the intervening process.

REFERENCES

1. HAMISTER, R. C. Test-retest reliability of the Wechsler Bellevue. *J. consult. Psychol.*, 1949, 13, 39–43.
2. JOHNSON, P. O. *Statistical Methods in Research.* New York: Prentice-Hall, 1949.

3. McNemar, Q. *Psychological Statistics.* New York: Wiley, 1949.
4. Slater, P. Interpreting Discrepancies. *Brit. J. Med. Psychol.* 1943, 19, 415–419.
5. U. S. Employment Service: *Guide to the use of General Aptitude Test Battery: Section III. Development.* Washington, D. C.: U. S. Dept. of Labor. 1955.
6. Wechsler, D. *The Measurement of Adult Intelligence.* (3rd ed.). Baltimore: Williams and Wilkins, 1944.

Part II

Applications in Assessment of Behavior

The most famous blind analysis in the psychological literature is that described by Osgood and Luria in the first paper of this section. Clinical psychologists very often complain of the barrenness of experimental approaches—a barrenness that is highlighted when they are brought face to face with the uniqueness of their patients. One would need very harsh standards of fertility to call the paper by Osgood and Luria, "barren." Indeed, so suited does the semantic differential as used by Osgood and Luria seem to the problems of the clinical psychologist that it is surprising that it has not become a more popular instrument with them. Some psychologists may be less fascinated by the dynamic interpretation that Osgood and Luria present than they are disappointed by the lack of any test of the predictions the authors made. Despite a certain incompleteness the paper remains, however, as a splendid example of how this particular technique can be used in the assessment of an individual patient.

One of the criticisms that may be made of the Repertory Grid technique which is described in the paper by Fransella and Adams is that an investigator must initially use whatever hunches he has to select relevant constructs and elements. But the problem of the investigator of individual cases, using instruments such as the Semantic Differential and the Repertory Grid technique, is no different from the problem of all scientists at the beginning of an investigation. All scientists must first of all take a chance in their selection of concepts, variables, units, and techniques when they embark on an investigation. Whether or not they have selected well can only be determined as the investigation proceeds. Once these things have been selected, however, and the investigation has started, the usual scientific requirement of objectivity is required. At the present time the Repertory Grid technique, at least as it is used in the investigation of individual cases, is perhaps a little too dependent on subjective interpretations. It would seem, however, that without too great a demand on our ingenuity it would be possible to incorporate into the technique a more objective quantitative aspect.

Scientific investigations must also, of course, be designed systematically and in such a way that their results are meaningful. Beech and Parboosingh, and Shapiro and Nelson, provide excellent examples of systematic approaches to patients' problems. The paper by Shapiro and Nelson demonstrates how cautious we must be in the assumptions we make about our measuring devices and how important it is to test, as far as possible, every one of our assumptions. The investigation reported by them also demonstrates how large group normative data obtained on the psychometric tests is required for the proper interpretation of the individual patient's responses. In general, their paper indicates that the distinction between individual and group studies is not firmly drawn.

Some clinicians often feel that the experimental approach necessitates complex apparatus, complicated statistics, or both. The final paper in this part in which Maryse Metcalfe describes a systematic investigation of a patient's asthmatic attacks clearly indicates that these are by no means necessary aspects of the experimental approach.

4

A Blind Analysis of a Case of Multiple Personality Using the Semantic Differential*

CHARLES E. OSGOOD and ZELLA LURIA

For more than a year the writers have been collecting semantic data from patients undergoing psychotherapy. This has been feasible through the cooperation of psychotherapists in various parts of the country. When the manuscript of "A Case of Multiple Personality" (*3*) arrived, the editor of this journal, without our knowledge, suggested to Thigpen and Cleckley that it would be interesting to have semantic data from each of the "personalities" in their patient. Thigpen and Cleckley accepted the suggestion and administered a form of the differential we have been using for this purpose to their patient in each of her three personalities. The editor also suggested that we might see how much these semantic data would allow us to infer about the patient without our having any knowledge of the case history, protocol, or prognosis. This appeared to be a useful and rather intriguing way to estimate the validity and sensitivity of this instrument. If we could infer descriptions of the three personalities which correspond with clinical observations, and if we could make reasonably accurate interpretations and predictions, we would be encouraged to continue our efforts to improve the semantic differential as a clinical tool.

---

* Reprinted from the *Journal of Abnormal and Social Psychology,* 1954, Vol. 49, pp. 579–591, by permission of the authors and the publisher.

THE SEMANTIC DIFFERENTIAL

The semantic differential is a combination of association and scaling procedures designed to give an objective measure of the connotative meaning of concepts. The underlying logic (*1*) can be summarized as follows: (*a*) The process of description or judgment can be conceived as the allocation of a concept to a set of experiential continua defined by pairs of polar terms. Thus the connotative meaning of a linguistically complex assertion, such as "My father has always been a rather submissive person," can be at least partially represented as

MY FATHER active__:__:__:__:X:__:__passive
MY FATHER soft__:X:__:__:__:__:__hard

The greater the strength of association, e.g., ". . . extremely submissive, a regular doormat," the more polarized, toward 1 or 7, the allocation (*2*). Since many scales of judgment are highly intercorrelated (e.g., *good-bad, fair-unfair, honest-dishonest, kind-cruel,* and so forth all reflect mainly the single "evaluative" factor in judgments), a limited number of such continua can be used to define a semantic space within which the connotative meaning of any concept can be specified. This clearly indicates some variant of factor analysis as the basic methodology in developing such an instrument. Two such analyses have been completed, both providing evidence for three general factors, "evaluation," "potency," and "activity," and some unknown number of specific factors that are probably denotative in nature.

The form of semantic differential we have been using in studying psychotherapy is based on this factor analytic work. In the 10 scales used, it gives approximately equal weight to the first three factors isolated. These scales and their factor loadings are given in Table 1. The 15 concepts used in this form of the differential were selected after consultation with clinicians and pretesting for their differentiating power. Ideally, they should sample the major persons and problems involved in therapy-in-general; we are not entirely satisfied with the present set, however, and more work should be done here. The concepts used are also shown in Table 1. In the test form itself, concepts are rotated against scales in such a way that each concept appears once with each scale, but with a maximum interval between successive appearances of both. The subject is instructed to do his checking rapidly, without struggling over particular items, to

TABLE 1

Concepts and Scales Used in This Analysis

Concepts

LOVE	MENTAL SICKNESS	SELF-CONTROL
CHILD	MY MOTHER	HATRED
MY DOCTOR	PEACE OF MIND	MY FATHER
ME	FRAUD	CONFUSION
MY JOB	MY SPOUSE	SEX

Scales and Their Factor Loadings

Scales	Evaluation	Activity	Potency
valuable-worthless	.79	.13	.04
clean-dirty	.82	.03	−.05
tasty-distasteful	.77	−.11	.05
fast-slow	.01	.70	.00
active-passive	.14	.59	.04
hot-cold	−.04	.46	−.06
large-small	.06	.34	.62
strong-weak	.19	.20	.62
deep-shallow	.27	.14	.46
tense-relaxed	−.55	.37	−.12

give his "immediate impressions." A 150-item form such as this usually takes less than 10 minutes to complete.

Reordering the raw data for a single subject on a single testing yields a matrix of N columns (here, 15 concepts) and i rows (here, 10 scales). The *meaning* of a particular concept to the subject, as defined by the operations of measurement here, is the profile of numbers in its column (or, more efficiently, the position in the n-dimensional space defined by the projection of these numbers onto the factors). *Difference in meaning* for two concepts is defined by the distance between their positions in this space as computed by the generalized distance formula, $D = \sqrt{\Sigma d^2}$, in which d is the difference in allocation of the two concepts on a single scale (*2*). The more similar any two concepts are in connotative meaning, the smaller will be the value of D. *Change in meaning* (of the same concept at different times during therapy, or in different "personalities") can be defined by the same operation, except that d here refers to the differences in allocation of the same concept on the same scale at different testings. The mathematical properties of this formula also allow us to represent the *semantic structure* of an individual in a concise form; computation of the distance, D, of every concept from every other concept yields an N/N matrix (here, 15/15) of distances which have the property of plotting within a space having dimensionality equal to the number of factors. To the extent that the individual subject being studied uses the same three factors isolated in our general factor work, his data will plot accurately in three dimensions.

THE SEMANTIC DATA

At this point we should state exactly what information we have about this case. We know that we are dealing with a case of triple personality, and these have been labeled for us (presumably by the therapists who collected the semantic data) "Eve White," "Eve Black," and "Jane." We suppose that the "White" and "Black" have some connotative significance—certainly, as will be seen, the quantitative semantic data distinguish sharply between them. We also know, of course, that the patient is a woman, presumably participating in some kind of therapy; we do not know the stage of therapy or whether or not she is hospitalized. We considered it also fair to ask (from J. McV. Hunt) about the following items of sociological status, because they contribute to the meaningful interpretation of certain concepts: Concept CHILD—does this woman have a child? Yes, she does. Concept SPOUSE—is this woman married? Yes, she is. Concepts FATHER and MOTHER—are her parents alive? The mother is, but Hunt doesn't know about the father. Concept MY JOB—has this woman had a job outside of homekeeping? Yes, she has.

This is the sum total of our external information about the case.

The semantic differential was given to this woman twice while "in" each of her three personalities; a period of about 2 months intervened between the two testings. The raw semantic data for each of the three personalities are given in Tables 2–4. The roman numerals I and II refer to first and second testings respectively.[2] We take the space to give these raw data in full so that anyone who is interested may study them and test any particular "hypotheses" about the case he wishes. Low values in these tables indicate judgments toward the polar term on the left and high values judgments toward the polar term on the right. The data in these tables show the semantic profiles, or meanings, of each concept at each testing and while "in" each personality. Since the form given at each testing was actually a double form (each item repeated once), we were able to estimate the reliability of these data. The immediate test-retest reliability coefficients for each of the testings are as follows: Eve White I, .82; Eve White II, .90; Eve Black I, .65; Eve Black II, .89; Jane I, .89; Jane II, .94. These coefficients indicate (*a*) a generally satisfactory level of reliability, (*b*) a consistent trend in all three personalities toward greater stability through time, and (*c*) that Jane is the most consistent or stable personality over short intervals of time and Eve Black is the least.

To obtain measures of semantic similarity and structure, we computed the matrices of *D* for each concept with every other concept, for each personality and testing. With an ordinary desk calculator and a table of square roots, these operations are very simple and rapid. In order to conserve space, the six matrices of *D* are not given here. These "distances" are based on application of the formula given earlier across all 10 scales. For convenience in plotting the models which appear as Figs. 1–6, the data for scales contributing to each of the three factors were averaged and new *D*'s computed. This, in effect, forces those data into three dimensions and, hence, into solid models that have no error. The very slight amount of distortion, or loss of information, resulting from this averaging process and restriction to three dimensions can be seen from the following correlations between original (10 scale) and "factor" *D* matrices (3 average scales): Eve White I, .91; Eve White II, .93; Eve Black I, .96; Eve Black II, .98; Jane I, .86; Jane II, .92. In other words, nearly all of the variance in this woman's judgments can be accounted for in terms of three factors. Figures 1–6, then, provide quite accurate representations of the ways various concepts are related in each of the personalities; the smaller the distance between any two concepts the more similar in connotative meaning they are.

THE THREE PERSONALITIES AND THEIR CHANGES THROUGH TIME

The general assumption we are following is that "mental illness" is essentially a disordering of meanings or ways of perceiving from those characteristic of people judged "normal" in our society, and that the process of psychotherapy from the patient's point of view is essentially a reordering and changing of these meanings. Within the limitations of our type of measurement and our sampling of concepts, the locations and relations among concepts shown in Figs. 1–6 can be thought of as pictures of how this woman perceives herself, the significant people about her, and certain modes of action—when functioning "in" her several personalities. We assume that this woman is receiving some kind of treatment through the period covered by our two samplings, I and II, and therefore look particularly for the types of changes in meaning that are taking place in the three personalities, as well as at the general nature of their organization. For purposes of ready comparison, all of the models are oriented in respect to the concept MY DOCTOR, which stays practically constant in meaning (*good, strong,* and *quite active*) through both time and personalities; spatially, in the figures, *good* is up and *bad* down, *active* to the left and *passive* to the right, and *strong* is away from the viewer while *weak* is near to or toward the viewer; the solid ball represents the origin of the space, e.g., a hypothetical "meaningless" concept that would result from checking all 4's.

Eve White

Semantic structures for Eve White I and II are shown in Figs. 1 and 2. The most general characterization would be that *Eve*

Fig. 1. Eve White I.

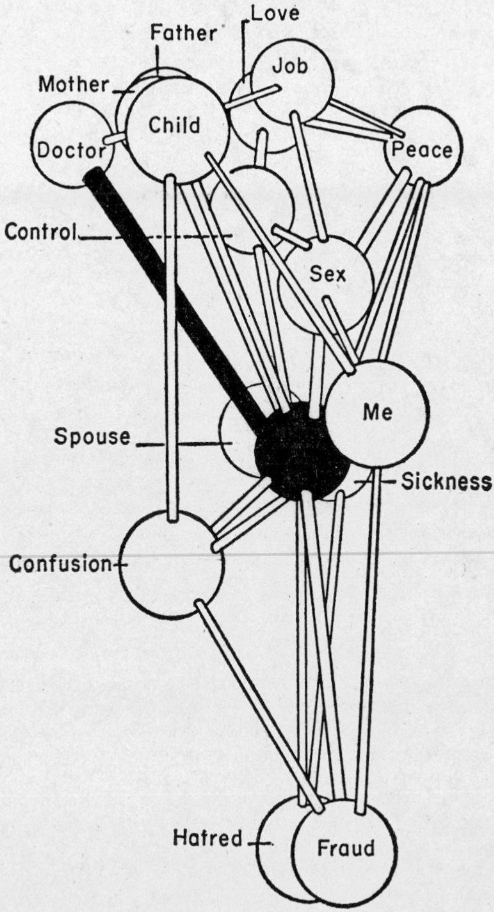

White perceives "the world" in an essentially normal fashion, is well socialized, but has an unsatisfactory attitude toward herself. Here the usual societal "goods" are seen favorably—MY DOCTOR, MY FATHER, LOVE, SELF-CONTROL, PEACE OF MIND, and MY MOTHER are all *good* and *strong* whereas FRAUD, HATRED, and to some extent CONFUSION are *bad*. The chief evidence of disturbance in the personality is the fact that ME (the self concept) is considered a little *bad,* a little *passive,* and definitely *weak.* Substantiating evidence is the *weakness* of her CHILD, as she sees him (or her), and the essential meaninglessness to her of MY

Fig. 2. Eve White II.

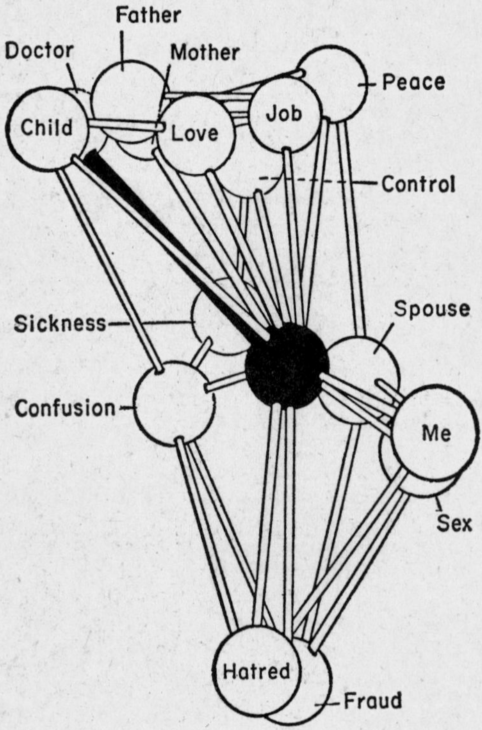

SPOUSE and SEX. Note also the wide evaluative separation between LOVE and SEX. In the interval between testings I and II ME and SEX become more *bad* and *passive* and simultaneously become almost identical in meaning to her—and note that her conceptions of LOVE (a good, strong thing) and SEX (a bad, weak thing like herself) have moved still further apart.

TABLE 2

Raw Data for Eve White

	LOVE		CHILD		MY DOCTOR		ME		MY JOB		MENTAL SICKNESS		MY MOTHER		PEACE OF MIND		FRAUD		MY SPOUSE		SELF-CONTROL		HATRED		MY FATHER		CON-FUSION		SEX		
	I	II	I	II	I	II	I	II	I	II	I	II	I	II	I	II	I	II	I	II	I	II	I	II	I	II	I	II	I	II	
cold	5.0	5.5	4.0	6.0	6.0	5.0	4.0	3.5	5.0	4.0	4.0	5.0	1.5	6.0	5.5	4.0	1.0	1.0	4.0	2.5	4.0	5.0	1.0	1.0	6.0	5.0	1.0	4.0	3.5	2.0	hot
valuable	1.0	1.0	1.0	1.0	1.0	1.0	4.0	6.0	1.0	1.0	1.0	4.0	1.0	1.0	1.0	1.0	7.0	7.0	3.0	3.5	1.0	1.0	7.0	7.0	1.0	1.0	3.0	5.5	2.5	4.5	worthless
tense	4.0	2.5	4.0	7.0	7.0	7.0	1.0	1.0	2.0	2.0	1.0	1.0	1.5	3.5	7.0	6.5	1.0	1.0	4.0	5.5	5.0	3.0	1.0	1.5	1.5	6.0	1.0	1.0	4.5	2.5	relaxed
small	7.0	6.0	1.0	7.0	7.0	7.0	1.0	2.0	5.5	6.5	7.0	6.5	5.5	7.0	7.0	7.0	1.0	1.0	5.0	5.5	6.5	6.5	1.0	1.0	7.0	7.0	7.0	5.0	6.0	2.5	large
fast	7.0	4.5	2.5	2.0	3.0	2.0	5.5	6.0	5.5	4.0	7.0	6.0	1.0	2.0	7.0	6.0	1.0	2.0	4.0	4.0	6.0	6.0	7.0	3.0	4.0	2.0	1.0	2.0	5.0	4.0	slow
dirty	7.0	7.0	7.0	7.0	7.0	7.0	5.5	6.0	7.0	7.0	5.5	6.5	7.0	7.0	7.0	7.0	1.0	1.0	5.0	4.5	5.0	6.5	1.0	1.0	7.0	7.0	1.5	6.0	5.5	3.0	clean
weak	7.0	5.0	1.0	1.0	7.0	7.0	1.0	1.0	5.5	6.0	1.0	3.0	7.0	6.5	7.0	7.0	1.0	1.0	4.0	3.5	7.0	6.0	1.0	1.0	7.0	7.0	1.0	1.5	4.0	2.5	strong
tasty	1.0	2.0	1.0	1.0	1.0	1.0	3.0	5.5	1.0	1.5	7.0	5.0	1.0	1.0	1.0	1.0	7.0	7.0	4.0	5.5	1.0	1.5	7.0	7.0	1.0	1.0	7.0	7.0	4.5	5.5	distasteful
deep	1.0	2.0	1.0	2.0	1.0	1.5	4.5	4.0	2.0	2.5	1.0	1.0	2.5	1.5	1.0	1.0	7.0	1.0	2.5	3.5	1.0	2.0	4.0	1.0	1.0	2.0	1.0	1.0	1.5	3.5	shallow
active	1.0	2.5	1.0	1.0	1.0	1.0	4.0	5.0	2.5	4.0	1.0	1.0	1.0	1.0	7.0	3.5	4.0	2.0	4.5	4.5	1.0	2.0	1.0	2.0	2.5	1.0	1.0	1.5	4.0	5.0	passive

TABLE 3

Raw Data for Eve Black

	LOVE		CHILD		MY DOCTOR		ME		MY JOB		MENTAL SICKNESS		MY MOTHER		PEACE OF MIND		FRAUD		MY SPOUSE		SELF-CONTROL		HATRED		MY FATHER		CON-FUSION		SEX		
	I	II	I	II	I	II	I	II	I	II	I	II	I	II	I	II	I	II	I	II	I	II	I	II	I	II	I	II	I	II	
cold	4.0	1.0	1.0	1.0	7.0	7.0	7.0	7.0	1.0	1.0	1.0	1.0	1.0	1.5	7.0	5.5	6.5	6.0	2.5	1.0	3.5	2.0	6.0	6.0	7.0	6.5	4.0	1.0	1.0	1.0	hot
valuable	7.0	7.0	7.0	6.0	1.0	1.0	1.0	1.0	7.0	7.0	7.0	7.0	4.5	2.5	1.0	3.0	2.0	2.0	7.0	7.0	4.5	4.5	1.5	2.0	1.0	1.0	7.0	7.0	7.0	7.0	worthless
tense	1.0	1.0	1.0	1.5	7.0	7.0	7.0	7.0	4.0	1.0	2.5	1.0	4.0	2.0	7.0	6.5	6.0	6.0	4.0	2.0	2.0	2.0	6.5	5.0	1.0	2.0	1.5	1.0	1.0	1.0	relaxed
small	1.0	1.0	7.0	1.0	7.0	7.0	4.0	7.0	5.5	1.0	4.0	1.0	4.0	4.5	7.0	5.5	6.5	6.5	2.5	1.0	6.0	4.5	6.5	6.0	1.0	4.0	4.0	1.0	1.0	1.0	large
fast	7.0	1.0	4.0	3.5	1.0	1.0	1.0	2.0	7.0	7.0	1.0	1.0	1.0	1.0	1.0	1.0	1.5	1.5	7.0	6.5	2.0	1.5	1.0	1.5	4.0	1.5	4.5	1.5	4.0	5.5	slow
dirty	2.0	2.0	1.0	3.0	7.0	7.0	7.0	7.0	4.0	1.0	1.5	1.0	7.0	4.0	7.0	6.0	5.0	6.0	4.0	1.0	4.5	4.5	6.0	6.5	7.0	7.0	1.5	1.0	4.0	1.0	clean
weak	1.0	1.0	7.0	1.5	7.0	7.0	7.0	7.0	1.0	1.0	1.0	1.0	4.0	7.0	7.0	6.0	6.0	6.0	4.0	1.0	5.0	5.0	6.5	6.0	1.0	4.0	1.0	1.0	1.0	1.0	strong
tasty	7.0	7.0	7.0	6.0	1.5	1.0	1.0	1.0	7.0	7.0	7.0	7.0	7.0	5.5	1.0	1.5	2.0	2.0	5.5	7.0	3.5	4.5	2.0	2.0	1.0	1.0	4.0	7.0	7.0	7.0	distasteful
deep	7.0	7.0	7.0	2.5	1.0	1.0	1.0	1.0	7.0	7.0	4.0	7.0	7.0	1.5	1.0	2.0	1.5	2.0	4.0	7.0	2.0	1.5	1.5	2.0	7.0	2.0	4.0	4.0	7.0	7.0	shallow
active	7.0	7.0	7.0	7.0	1.0	1.0	1.0	1.0	7.0	7.0	7.0	7.0	1.0	1.0	1.0	1.0	1.5	1.5	7.0	7.0	4.5	4.0	1.5	1.5	1.0	1.0	4.0	7.0	7.0	7.0	passive

TABLE 4

Raw Data for Jane

	LOVE		CHILD		MY DOCTOR		ME		MY JOB		MENTAL SICKNESS		MY MOTHER		PEACE OF MIND		FRAUD		MY SPOUSE		SELF-CONTROL		HATRED		MY FATHER		CON-FUSION		SEX		
	I	II	I	II	I	II	I	II	I	II	I	II	I	II	I	II	I	II	I	II	I	II	I	II	I	II	I	II	I	II	
cold	4.0	6.0	4.0	6.5	4.0	6.5	4.0	5.5	4.0	6.0	4.0	4.0	4.5	4.5	4.0	6.5	1.0	2.0	4.0	6.0	4.0	6.0	1.0	1.5	6.0	6.5	4.0	4.5	4.0	6.5	hot
valuable	1.0	1.0	1.0	1.0	1.0	1.0	4.0	2.0	1.0	1.0	2.0	2.0	1.0	1.0	1.0	1.0	7.0	7.0	4.0	1.0	1.0	1.0	6.0	7.0	1.0	1.0	2.5	4.0	1.0	1.0	worthless
tense	7.0	7.0	5.0	5.0	7.0	7.0	2.0	1.0	1.5	2.0	1.0	1.0	1.5	2.0	7.0	7.0	1.5	2.0	7.0	7.0	7.0	6.5	1.0	1.5	1.5	2.0	1.0	1.5	7.0	7.0	relaxed
small	7.0	7.0	7.0	6.5	7.0	7.0	4.0	4.5	7.0	6.5	7.0	6.5	5.5	6.5	7.0	7.0	4.5	1.5	7.0	7.0	7.0	7.0	4.5	2.0	7.0	7.0	6.0	4.0	6.5	7.0	large
fast	7.0	6.5	3.0	1.5	1.0	2.0	4.5	2.0	7.0	7.0	7.0	6.0	3.5	2.0	7.0	6.0	1.5	2.0	3.0	2.5	7.0	6.0	7.0	4.0	2.0	2.0	1.5	2.0	4.0	4.0	slow
dirty	7.0	7.0	7.0	7.0	7.0	7.0	7.0	7.0	7.0	7.0	7.0	7.0	7.0	7.0	7.0	7.0	1.0	2.0	7.0	7.0	7.0	7.0	2.0	2.0	7.0	7.0	7.0	4.0	7.0	7.0	clean
weak	7.0	7.0	4.0	6.0	7.0	7.0	4.5	4.0	6.5	6.5	4.0	5.0	2.0	6.0	7.0	7.0	1.0	2.0	7.0	7.0	7.0	7.0	1.0	2.0	7.0	7.0	4.0	4.0	7.0	6.5	strong
tasty	1.0	1.0	1.0	1.0	1.0	1.0	3.5	2.0	4.5	2.0	5.0	4.0	2.0	1.0	1.0	1.0	7.0	7.0	1.0	1.0	1.0	1.0	7.0	7.0	1.0	1.0	7.0	5.5	1.0	1.0	distasteful
deep	1.0	1.0	1.0	2.0	1.0	1.5	2.0	3.0	1.0	1.5	1.0	1.5	1.0	2.0	1.0	1.5	1.0	2.0	2.0	2.0	1.0	1.5	1.0	2.0	1.0	1.5	1.0	1.5	4.0	1.0	shallow
active	2.5	1.5	1.0	1.0	1.0	1.0	2.0	1.5	4.5	2.0	1.0	1.0	1.0	1.0	5.5	2.5	6.0	4.5	4.0	1.0	2.5	2.0	2.5	2.0	1.0	1.0	1.5	2.5	4.0	1.5	passive

Eve Black

Semantic structures for Eve Black I and II are shown in Figs. 3 and 4. The most general characterization here would be that *Eve Black has achieved a violent kind of adjustment in which she perceives herself as literally perfect, but, to accomplish this break, her way of perceiving "the world" becomes completely disoriented from the norm.* The only exceptions to this dictum

Fig. 3. Eve Black I.

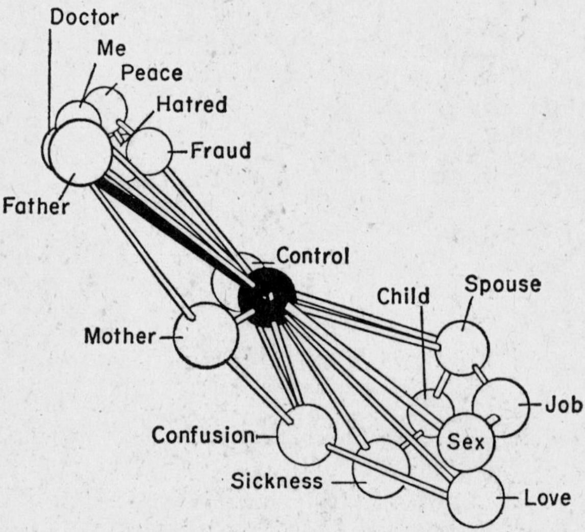

are MY DOCTOR and PEACE OF MIND, which maintain their *good* and *strong* characteristics, the latter, interestingly enough, also becoming *active* on II. But if Eve Black perceives herself as being *good,* then she also has to accept HATRED and FRAUD as positive values, since (we assume) she has strong hatreds and is socially fraudulent. So we find a tight, but very un-normal, favorable cluster of ME, MY DOCTOR, PEACE OF MIND, HATRED, and FRAUD. What are positive values for most people—CHILD, MY SPOUSE, MY JOB, LOVE, and SEX—are completely rejected as *bad* and *passive,* and all of these except CHILD are also *weak* (this may be because CHILD was weak in Eve White and much

Fig. 4. Eve Black II.

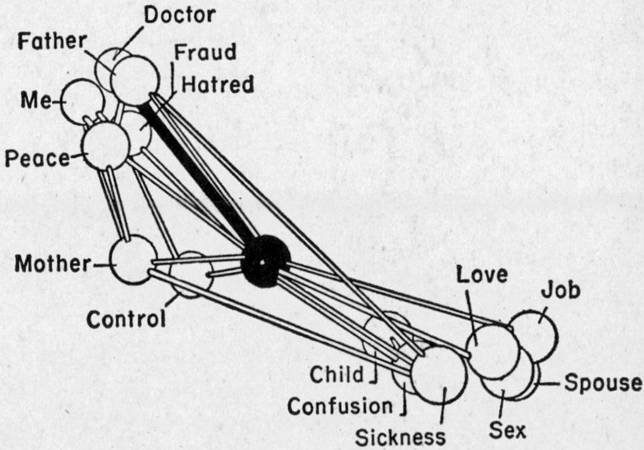

of the change here is a simple "flip-flop" of meanings). Note that it is MOTHER in this personality that becomes relatively meaningless; FATHER, on the other hand, stays *good* but shifts completely from *strong* (in Eve White) to *weak*—possible implications of these familial identifications will be considered later. Note also that in this personality LOVE and SEX are closely identified, both as *bad, weak, passive* things.

Jane

Semantic structures for Jane I and II are shown in Figs. 5 and 6. The general characterization is that *Jane displays the most "healthy" meaning pattern, in which she accepts the usual evaluations of concepts by her society yet still maintains a satisfactory evaluation of herself.* MY FATHER, MY MOTHER, MY CHILD, and MY DOCTOR—most of the significant persons in her life—are seen as *good, strong,* and *active.* The major modes of behavior, PEACE OF MIND, LOVE, SELF-CONTROL, and MY JOB, are seen as equally *good* and *strong,* but *somewhat passive*—as if these ways of behaving and thinking were simply accepted without stress. The two socially agreed-upon evils, HATRED and FRAUD, are put in their proper places. The most significant characteristics of

Jane's meaning system, however, are these: The self concept, ME, while still not *strong* (but not *weak*, either) is nearer the *good* and *active* directions of the semantic space; note also the close identification of ME and MENTAL SICKNESS, which here is

Fig. 5. Jane I.

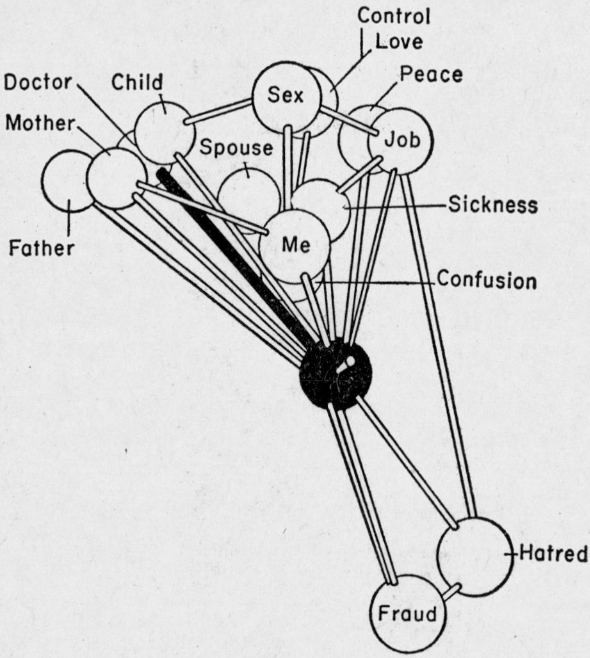

not an unfavorable concept to her. Her attitude toward her husband, MY SPOUSE, is for the first time meaningful (unlike Eve White) and tending toward the *good, strong, active* directions, like the other significant persons (unlike Eve Black). And LOVE and SEX (quite unlike Eve White) are both favorable and quite closely identified. The changes from testings I to II are simply such as to strengthen the "healthy" pattern evident in the first view. ME becomes considerably more *good* and *active;* MY SPOUSE for the first time becomes completely identified connotatively with MY DOCTOR and MY FATHER (and loses its tie with

Fig. 6. Jane II.

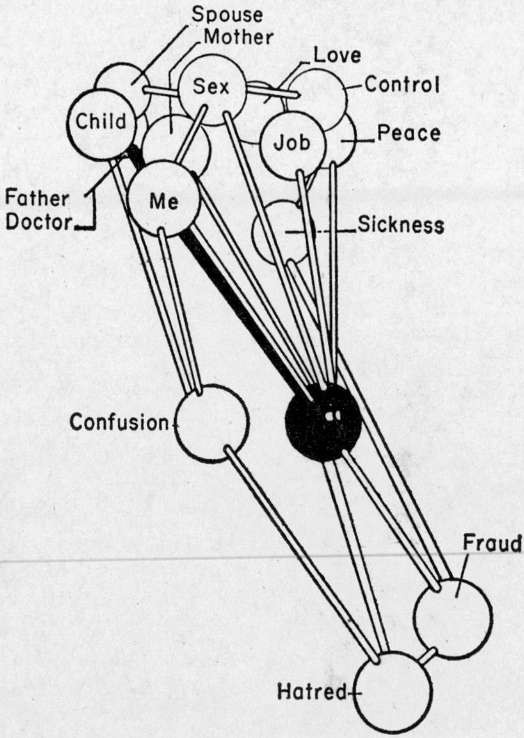

CONFUSION); and LOVE and SEX become intimately identified with each other and close in meaning to SELF-CONTROL and PEACE OF MIND.

The thumbnail semantic sketches of each personality just given make it intuitively evident that the semantic differential does draw sharp distinctions between the three personalities inhabiting one nervous system. It is possible to demonstrate these distinctions quantitatively by intercorrelating *D* matrices between personalities and over time. If two of our models are generally similar in structure, such that large and small distances between concepts in one are reflected also in the other, then the *r* will be high. Table 5 gives these correlations. The first thing to note is

TABLE 5

Correlations of D-Matrices between Personalities and over Time

	White I	White II	Black I	Black II	Jane I	Jane II
White I	—					
White II	.73	—				
Black I	−.06	—	—			
Black II	—	−.02	.86	—		
Jane I	.73	—	−.26	—	—	
Jane II	—	.53	—	−.08	.92	—

that the correlation of each personality with itself (e.g., testings I and II) is regularly much higher than the correlation of that personality with any other personality (with the single exception of Eve White I and Jane I). This is quantitative justification for the statement that the semantic differential does differentiate between the several personalities of this woman. Whether it differentiates in a valid way is a matter that can be judged only by relating our analysis to the detailed case history material available elsewhere (*3*).

Another important thing to note about these correlations is that Eve White and Jane (the two "socialized" personalities) are fairly highly correlated whereas the correlations of Eve Black with the other two are definitely low, even negative. In other words, Eve Black is clearly the most deviant and disordered personality. Finally, it should be noted that these three personalities differ somewhat in their stability, as indexed by the I/II correlations, Eve White being the least stable and Jane the most.

CHANGES IN MEANING OF SPECIFIC CONCEPTS

As noted earlier, the meaning of a specific concept is operationally defined as its profile against the differential (e.g., its position in semantic space). Change in meaning between testings I and II can be measured directly by the *D* between I and II profiles for the same concept (e.g., between the paired columns in

Tables 2–4). These *D* values are given under "Within Personalities, Between Testings" in Table 6. Changes in meaning between

TABLE 6

Changes in Meaning of Specific Concepts

Concept	Within Personalities, Between Testings			Between Personalities, Within Testings					
	$D_{I\text{-}II}$ Eve White	$D_{I\text{-}II}$ Eve Black	$D_{I\text{-}II}$ Jane	$D_{W\text{-}B}$		$D_{W\text{-}J}$		$D_{B\text{-}J}$	
				I	II	I	II	I	II
LOVE	.42	.67	.23	1.58	1.44	.35	.57	1.62	1.81
CHILD	.71	.96	.37	1.65	1.40	.68	.54	1.47	1.41
MY DOCTOR	.15	.05	.27	.23	.23	.28	.25	.30	.12
ME	.36	.32	.42	1.21	1.40	*.60*	*.88*	.83	.77
MY JOB	.27	.62	.42	1.30	1.43	.49	.43	1.19	1.54
MENTAL SICKNESS	.45	.45	.19	1.24	1.38	.40	.32	1.30	1.47
MY MOTHER	.54	.78	.46	.71	.78	.66	.23	1.02	.68
PEACE OF MIND	.40	.35	.41	.86	.66	.21	.28	.81	.61
FRAUD	.64	.12	.40	1.46	1.35	*.73*	.34	1.29	1.22
MY SPOUSE	.30	.62	.47	.67	.96	*.61*	*.89*	1.04	1.75
SELF-CONTROL	.32	.25	.24	.78	.80	.34	.39	.92	1.01
HATRED	.51	.19	.44	1.54	1.31	.51	.23	1.37	1.19
MY FATHER	.53	.71	.09	1.06	.60	.25	.43	1.06	.43
CONFUSION	.64	.67	.44	.86	.96	.71	.42	.98	.88
SEX	.62	.34	.47	1.10	.62	*.63*	*1.20*	1.45	1.76

Note.—Numbers in italics indicate concepts that serve best to characterize differences between Eve White and Jane.

personalities for the same concepts can be measured directly by the *D* between profiles for the same concept but as judged in two different personalities; these *D* values are given under "Between Personalities, Within Testings" in Table 6.

Semantic Stability Through Time

In general, although the differences are not great, Eve Black is the least stable personality through time and Jane the most stable (cf., columns 2–4 in Table 6). The concept-by-concept data thus confirm the stability of Jane as shown in the structural data given above. For Eve White the most unstable or labile concepts are CHILD, MY MOTHER, FRAUD, HATRED, MY FATHER, CONFUSION, and SEX. For Eve Black the most labile concepts are LOVE, CHILD, MY JOB, MY MOTHER, MY SPOUSE, MY FATHER, and CONFUSION. For Jane the most unstable notions are ME, MY JOB, MY MOTHER, MY SPOUSE, HATRED, CONFUSION, and SEX. We note that the family constellation—mother, father, spouse, child—tend to be more susceptible to change through time within these personalities, but that the self concept stays relatively constant within personalities (e.g., the location of the self concept, in a sense, defines these three personalities). HATRED, SEX, and CONFUSION also seem to be points of stress.

Semantic Stability Between Personalities

The data given in columns 5–10 in Table 6 make it clear that concept meanings in general shift more between Eve Black and the other two than between Jane and Eve White, this again substantiating the over-all correlations between total structures. The only concept that remains strictly constant in meaning through the personality changes in this woman is MY DOCTOR, although PEACE OF MIND and CONFUSION show greater stability than most others. It is interesting to note which concepts serve best to characterize the differences between Eve White and Jane (Eve Black shows gross differences on almost all concepts). These two "socialized" personalities differ from one another chiefly on ME, MY SPOUSE, and SEX, and these differences are increasing in magnitude through time. This clearly suggests this woman's sexual life as a core problem, Eve White being highly critical of all three concepts and Jane accepting them as positive values. It is also interesting to note in this connection that semantic differences between Eve White and Jane on CHILD, MY MOTHER, FRAUD, HATRED, and CONFUSION are decreasing through time.

INTERPRETATIONS OF THESE SEMANTIC DATA

The analyses of these personalities and their changes given so far have been descriptive rather than interpretive for the most part. In a sense, we have merely put into words what this woman herself, in her several personalities, has indicated by her check marks. The treatment of semantic differential data, from the patterns of check marks to construction of the models shown in Figs. 1–6, is completely objective, and any investigator starting from the same data and following the rules would have to end up with the same pictures we have.

Making interpretations and predictions about this case on a "blind" basis is another matter entirely. In this section we go far beyond the objective data, and we are consequently much less confident about our statements. For one thing, neither of the writers is an experienced clinician—certainly not experienced with respect to the dynamics and characteristics of multiple personality. For another thing, we do not know at what stage in therapy our two testings were made, and interpretation would certainly vary greatly in terms of such information. It should also be pointed out that in the ordinary use of the semantic differential as a clinical tool (as compared with a blind analysis) many other sources of information would be available to support certain alternative interpretations and render others farcical. Let it be understood, then, that what follows is a flight into conjecture, in contrast with the preceding, factual reporting of semantic data.

Interpretive Descriptions of the Three Personalities

Eve White is the woman who is simultaneously most in contact with social reality and under the greatest emotional stress. She is aware of both the demands of society and her own inadequacies in meeting them. She sees herself as a passive weakling and is also consciously aware of the discord in her sexual life, drawing increasingly sharp distinctions between LOVE as an idealized notion and SEX as a crude reality. She maintains the greatest diversity among the meanings of various concepts. She is concerned and ambivalent about her CHILD, but apparently is *not* aware of her own ambivalent attitudes toward her MOTHER—and seems to become more resistant to this by testing II. Those psychoanalytically inclined may wish to identify Eve White with dominance of the *superego:* certainly, the superego seems to view the world through the eyes of Eve White, accepting the mores or values of others (particularly her mother) but continuously criticizing and punishing herself. If this case came to the psychotherapists with a voluntary, self-initiated plea for help, then it seems likely that Eve White was dominant at the time.

Eve Black is clearly the most out of contact with social reality and simultaneously the most self-assured. To rhapsodize, Eve Black finds PEACE OF MIND through close identification with a God-like therapist (MY DOCTOR, probably a father symbol for her), accepting her HATRED and FRAUD as perfectly legitimate aspects of the God-like role. Naturally, she sees herself as a dominant, active wonder-woman and is in no way self-critical. She is probably unaware of her family situation. Those psychoanalytically inclined could say that the *id* looks out at the world through the eyes of Eve Black. Like a completely selfish infant, this personality is entirely oriented around the assumption of its own perfection. Actually, Eve Black seems to be more harmonious with the Adlerian than with the Freudian model, since personal perfection is apparently the demand acceded to rather than sexuality. If the case was committed to an institution, it seems likely that this personality was the reason for commitment.

Jane is the most puzzling of the three personalities, and our interpretation will have to depend upon assumptions about the stage of treatment (see below). Superficially, Jane is a very healthy personality: "all's well with the world, and day by day I'm getting better and better." Thus we find all the people in her life perceived as *good* and *strong* and *active* and all the socially approved modes of action perceived as *good* and *strong* and *passive;* SEX is LOVE-ly, her SPOUSE is becoming more like the noble DOCTOR all the time, and she is coming to perceive herself even, as a pleasant and reasonably active (if somewhat weak and submissive) person. But all this is a little too rosy, a little too pat. We note that Jane is becoming more and more "simple-minded"—all of her judgments tending to fall along a single factor of *good-strong* vs. *bad-weak*—which makes the Jane II model the most restricted and undiversified of all. Those psychoanalytically inclined may wish to view this personality as representing dominance of a self-deceptive *ego* which has woven a web of repression as to the state of reality; or, they may wish to view Jane as an essentially strong, healthy, and improving ego-dominated personality. In any case, we doubt if Jane would have either come for therapy or have been institutionalized—as such.

Possible Dynamisms Operating in the Case

Identification mechanisms. We say the patient "identifies" with some other person when her meaning of herself, ME, is semantically close to her meaning of the other person; e.g., if she sees her father as a kind, active, relaxed, etc. person and describes herself in the same terms, we infer identification. However, the pattern of identifications displayed by this patient seems unusual. Only in Eve Black, the obviously disoriented personality in terms of her values, is there clear differential identification—with her FATHER (and this may reflect the semantic tie-up between FATHER and MY DOCTOR). Jane shows some slight tendency toward closer identification with MOTHER, but it is not close. Eve White shows none with either parent. The fact that identification with FATHER (and MY DOCTOR) in Eve Black is accompanied by rejection of MOTHER to meaninglessness is suggestive of an underlying conflict in identifications. Note also, in this connection, that in Eve Black I the ascendancy of ME to the *good, strong, active* position is accompanied by making FATHER *weak*—as if she were taking over her father's role and putting her mother in her own previous place. And, interestingly enough, the concept SELF-CONTROL suffers the same fate as MOTHER. This picture of Eve Black is certainly suggestive of an *Electra complex* as the underlying dynamism. In "real" life, her MOTHER is or was the dominant, threatening figure—moralizing, demanding standards and SELF-CONTROL—and in Eve Black this woman escapes the pressure by rendering both MOTHER and SELF-CONTROL meaningless and simultaneously identifying with and taking her FATHER's place (via the therapist). Suggestive evidence may be found in Tables 2–4: MOTHER is consistently *colder* than FATHER and usually more *tense* and *fast* (e.g., Factor 3). Identification of the self with the therapist in Eve Black is perfect, of course. The concept MY DOCTOR is the only personal concept to show perfect stability both between personalities and through time. The patient thus displays what might be called maximal *positive transference* in all three personalities; there is no sign of any negative transference at either testing, which may be indicative of the stage of therapy (e.g., early).

Significance of the patient's sexual life. Although Jane shows a rosy acceptance of normal sexual patterning—with LOVE and SEX linked and passively favorable, Eve White clearly displays awareness of a basic conflict in this area—SEX is early somewhat more distasteful than LOVE and becomes distinctly distasteful and dirty by testing II. In Eve White also we find ME and MY SPOUSE becoming linked with sex in this unpleasant location. Eve Black, on the other hand, rejects both SEX and LOVE—but closely links them in her thinking. If we were to relate these facts with the Electra situation described above, the interpretation would be that her persisting conflict with her mother and attempts to identify with her father make it impossible for her to experience normal sexual satisfactions with her husband and to carry out the normal mother-wife-home role. Eve White is aware of this, in a sense, but Jane clearly is not. The concept MY JOB is interesting in this connection: its persistent linkages with LOVE, PEACE OF MIND, and SELF-CONTROL in the two "socialized" personalities, coupled with its linkage with SEX and MY SPOUSE in Eve Black, clearly suggests to us that this woman is interpreting MY JOB in the sense of "my job as a mother, wife, and homebuilder" rather than in terms of her outside work (which we understand she has). In any case, there is clear evidence of involvement with her sex life as a major problem, and this may have been the presenting problem when she began therapy.

Repression and amnesia. Knowing that we are dealing with a case of multiple personality—usually characterized by complete dissociation between states—it is interesting to speculate on what meanings are repressed in the several personalities. It will be recalled that, operationally, meaninglessness of a concept is defined by its closeness to the origin (the solid balls in the models). This is probably to be interpreted as "connotative deadness" or "damping of affect" with respect to the concept involved. Within the matrix of our instrument, however, there is another way in which repression or amnesia may show up, and that is via a complete shift in meaning of the concept being judged (e.g., CHILD may shift from the personal reference of "my own youngster" to "children-in-general"). Looking back at the semantic data with these points in mind, we hazard the following guesses: Eve White probably has the best contact with reality and may not be amnesic at all (except for the other personalities); Eve Black may be amnesic for her mother and her own role as a mother and wife; Jane in Pollyanna fashion may be amnesic for her own problems, e.g., MENTAL SICKNESS and CONFUSION, and the indiscriminate way in which she lumps all socially favorable concepts at least suggests that she is judging CHILD, MOTHER, etc. in the abstract rather than as MY CHILD, MY MOTHER, and so forth.

Interpretation I—Assumed Early Stage of Therapy

The "original" personality, in the sense of being most characteristic of the woman her friends and relations knew, was Jane. The first testing of this personality shows a relatively weak ME that is associated with MENTAL SICKNESS; i.e., she was dimly aware of her own inadequacies but was striving to maintain a rigid acceptance of the real world and maintain an adequate home life. The people about her, with the exception of her husband, were seen as strong and active (perhaps threatening) in relation to herself, and her love life was regarded as a sort of deliberate, controlled duty. She was completely unaware of her (repressed) emotional ambivalence toward her mother, husband, and child. The things being hidden in this personality, and providing the force behind the eventual split, were (*a*) her Electra complex, (*b*) her repugnance for sexual relations with her husband, and (*c*) her ambivalent attitude toward herself. We suspect that she had a position in society that demanded "good front."

We must assume strong and about equal pressures toward solving the Electra complex, (*a*) by identifying with FATHER and asserting the self (id?), and (*b*) toward solving it by identifying with MOTHER and devaluing herself (superego?). This produces a two-way split away from the Jane pattern, one into Eve Black where selfish needs for superiority and playing the father role are achieved and another into Eve White where societal needs for submission and playing the mother role are achieved. This split, and the subsequent availability of the other roles, allows Jane to shift toward the "sweetness and light" view of the world, and this is clearly demonstrated by the changes between Jane I and Jane II. Eve White continues to become more simply and rigidly self-critical and Eve Black continues to become more simply and rigidly self-satisfied.

Assuming successful therapy is possible—which seems questionable—it will involve less and less time being spent in being Jane and Eve Black and a consequent shift into Eve White, where better contact and differentiation seems to be maintained. But here it will be necessary to bring Eve White to understand the reason for her depression, the role of her ambivalence toward her mother in her problem—which shows no signs of happening yet—and thence a gradual restructuring in which ME becomes more favorable, along with SPOUSE and SEX, and identifications with FATHER and MOTHER are reassigned. This will probably involve a period of negative transference, with MY DOCTOR and MOTHER becoming closely identified and being temporarily shifted to *bad, strong,* and *active* directions of the semantic space. In other words, successful treatment will mean increasing time spent in, and a gradual restructuring of, Eve White to the point where it incorporates what is now Jane, but with a realignment of significant persons. On the other hand, if this woman is in a mental institution and remains there, it seems likely that Eve Black will become the dominant house she lives in. In either case, it is probable that Jane will appear less and less.

Interpretation II—Assumed Late Stage of Therapy

If we assume that we are seeing the terminal stages of therapy with a case of this sort, then a quite different interpretation is necessary. The difference in interpretations hinges upon Jane, either as a deceptive and vanishing original personality (interpretation I) or as an increasingly healthy and augmenting personality (interpretation II). In the latter case we would assume that Eve White had been the "original" personality as people knew her—a socially acceptable wife and mother, but one laden with conflicts, anxieties, and self-criticism. The split in this case —into one personality in which the self-criticism completely disappears via irrationality (Eve Black) and another in which self-criticism vanishes via rationality (Jane)—seems less sensible, however. Jane seems unnecessary at this stage and really should have developed out of Eve White rather than being contemporaneous. If we assume there was a split in any case, Jane is clearly the most healthy personality, since LOVE and SEX are identified, the world is viewed in acceptable fashion, and the self concept is becoming more favorable all the time. The prediction here would be increasing time spent in Jane and less in the others. The stumbling blocks in the way of this interpretation are (*a*) the lack of any realignment of the system of parental identifications, and (*b*) the fact that Jane is becoming *less* diversified semantically (more "simple-minded") rather than the reverse. This second interpretation was actually the one we first adopted—because of the superficial "healthiness" of Jane—but consideration of all the evidence seems to favor the first interpretation. However, it should be noted that *if* this case is near the end of successful therapy, Jane is the only personality that combines both a normal view of the world and reasonable (increasing) acceptance of the self.

Interpretation III—Combination of I and II

It is possible to combine interpretations I and II by assuming that Jane is both the original personality which broke apart and the terminal personality which is being developed out of therapy. In this case, the early development of the case, probably in childhood, would be the same as that given under interpretation I—the conflicting parental identifications (id and superego determined respectively) were of about equal strength and finally became too intense to be contained within the self-deceptive personality organization of Jane. During the middle course of the case, when therapy was undertaken, we thus find all three personalities oscillating, temporary dominance of the mother and wife role being represented by Eve White, temporary dominance of the self-gratifying father role being represented by Eve Black, and temporary dominance of the face-saving, problem-solving ego being represented by Jane. Intentionally or unintentionally, the effect of therapy may be to strengthen the self-deceptive organization of Jane without resolving the underlying conflicts dramatized by Eve White and Eve Black. The oversimplified, Pollyanna-like ways of perceiving herself as *good* along with all the other significant persons in her life yields a superficially happy person who views the world in an acceptable, if rigidly stereotyped, fashion. If the present combined interpretation approximates the actual situation, then we feel compelled to predict another breakdown at some later period in this person's life. In other words, the effect of therapy (whatever type it may have been) seems to have been further to strengthen the self-deceptive original organization of Jane, while making this personality even more rigid and insensitive to subtle differences in meaning and without resolving the underlying conflicts which created the original disturbance.

What Price Therapy?

It is impossible to tell from our semantic data whether the increasing simplification in structure characteristic of all three personalities is due to therapy itself or is happening despite therapy. However, a number of specialists in psychotherapy have from time to time expressed concern over the "hidden" effects of therapy even in so-called successful cases—particularly reduction in initiative, creativeness, and flexibility of the patient. Certainly in the present case we are witnessing an over-all reduction in differentiation of meanings. If overt behavior is in considerable part determined by meanings, as we believe it is, then we must expect Jane (if she is the terminal personality) to be now even less capable of behaving differentially to her mother, father, spouse, and child—they are all essentially undifferentiated "strong-active-goodness" to her. This would also be true, but to a lesser extent, of Eve White, although here we would assume an earlier stage of therapy and hence a possibility of secondary elaboration of semantic diversity under sensitive therapy.

Is rigidity of this sort a necessary price of therapy? In striving to achieve the goals of societal acceptability and individual happiness, does the therapist have to sacrifice the richness, individuality, and subtler adjustiveness of the patient? These are serious questions raised by the data of this single case—but not answered by them, of course. From the larger sample of cases we are presently working on, better answers may be forthcoming, but the cases are generally less severe. One other interesting phenomenon in the present cases should be mentioned: Despite the gross changes in meaning of concepts in the several personalities, and the over-all reduction in diversity, the semantic judgmental frame of reference remains constant. In other words, all three of the personalities in this woman utilize semantic scales in the same ways—the correlations between scales are the same for all three personalities and reduction in diversity in all of them is accomplished by a coalescence of *good, strong,* and *active* into a single evaluative dimension. Thus it would appear that the level of scale meanings is below that at which concepts vary, and common to all three personalities.

REFERENCES

1. OSGOOD, C. E. The nature and measurement of meaning. *Psychol. Bull.,* 1952, *49,* 192–237.
2. OSGOOD, C. E., and SUCI, G. J. A measure of relation determined by both mean difference and profile information. *Psychol. Bull.,* 1952, *49,* 251–262.
3. THIGPEN, C. H., and CLECKLEY, H. A case of multiple personality. *J. abnorm. soc. Psychol.,* 1954, *49,* 135–151.

5

An Illustration of the Use of Repertory Grid Technique in a Clinical Setting*

FAY FRANSELLA and B. ADAMS

A modification of repertory grid technique has been used to study a man who had committed several acts of arson. Six grids of different types were given showing its flexibility and, within the limits of the sample of constructs used, that the technique has internal, predictive and content validity and indications of an acceptable level of test-retest reliability. These generalizations are true in spite of element changes but only so long as the elements are within the range of convenience of the constructs. Its possible uses include the testing of hypotheses derived from explanations of the behaviour of the individual patient, a method of tracing conceptual changes in the patient resulting from psychotherapy and a possible basis for the development of a measure of prognosis.

INTRODUCTION

The history of psychiatric ideas concerning fire-raising shows that the concept was more narrowly defined in the past than it is today. Marc (1833) classified fire-raisers under the diagnosis *monomania* and they became the centre of legal and psychiatric controversy regarding responsibility under law. In England Pritchard (1822) included these people under the general term *moral insanity* thus partially avoiding legal issues since they were rarely considered certifiably insane. In America at this time views were more in agreement with those of today and Pilgrim (1884) de-

* Reprinted from the *British Journal of Social and Clinical Psychology*, 1966, Vol. 5, pp. 51–62, by permission of the authors and the publisher.

nied that pyromania was a psychological entity stating that it was "either a crime or the symptom of a disease or ill-developed brain." Later writers examined the psychopathology in more detail and traced out three groups of fire-raisers; children performing it as an aggressive act, similar acts in the mentality subnormal and a group in which it was associated with sexual activity.

Lewis & Yarnell (1951) showed that in a group of fire-raisers, from which were excluded only those in whom intent to defraud was established, all psychiatric diagnostic groups were represented. In an attempt to trace common factors which preceded the acts of arson they concluded that the majority "had allowed themselves to be pressurized into a state of tension and despair by an accumulation of unhappy events . . . just prior to the fire-setting there was a fear that if something drastic did not happen their whole personality was going to explode and disintegrate." Although this describes the mental state at the time, it fails to account for the selection of fire-raising as an act, or to indicate what function this behaviour might have.

Assertions as to the meaning of fire to fire-raisers have, in the past, been made on a speculative basis and have concerned fire-raisers in general. The purpose of the present study is to illustrate how, using a recently developed technique (the Repertory Grid), statements about the meaning of fire can be based on test evidence and made specific to a particular individual. In so doing it is intended to demonstrate some of the ways in which repertory grid technique can be used to elicit information and test hypotheses about a patient's thinking behaviour.

RELEVANT PERSONAL HISTORY

The patient, a married shopkeeper of 39, was the eldest of four siblings in a closely-knit Presbyterian family whose home was a small Scots industrial village. There was no evidence of psychiatric illness in the family. His personality was characterized by extreme conscientiousness and dislike of change, he possessed considerable drive and strongly held opinions regarding sexual and business morality. Eighteen months before admission he commenced acts of arson and later described how tense and aggressive feelings would be relieved temporarily by the calmness which immediately followed the fire-setting. After being charged he admitted nine episodes in all and was sentenced to a term of imprisonment and subsequently referred to the Maudsley Hospital.

REPERTORY GRID TECHNIQUE

A variety of versions of repertory grid technique have been developed since it was first described by Kelly (1955). Certain aspects of the development of the technique have been outlined by Bannister (1962) and the basic scoring procedure used in this study is that described by Bannister (1963).

Two terms basic to the technique are (i) *elements:* these are the "stimulus-objects" it is the subject's task to rank order in terms of (ii) *constructs:* these are dimensions used by a person in conceptualizing aspects of his world. Constructs can be elicited or supplied and Kelly describes a method for eliciting by presenting the subject with three of the elements and asking him to "name some important way in which two of these are alike and thereby different from the third." The criterion for selection of elements is that they should be within the *range of convenience* of the constructs, i.e. they should be relevant to the constructs.

Method

The elements, ten in each case, were presented to the subject and a card with the words of a construct such as "like me in character" was shown to him. The subject's task was to select the element (e.g. the person) which is most like him in character and to rank in order the remaining people down to the one who is least like him in character.

Scoring

A rank order correlation matrix is constructed and the Spearman rho's are calculated for each construct with every other construct. Since correlations are not linear, the squares of the rho's multiplied by 100 are used as scores and the score is in effect the "percentage variance in common" between any two constructs. A total of the matrix relationships for construct one can be worked out by adding the squares of the rho's times 100 for that construct with all others, e.g. $1 - 2 + 1 - 3 + 1 - 4 \ldots + 1 - n$.

The construct with this highest total score is extracted as the major axis and the second axis is that construct with the next highest total score which is not significantly correlated (for practical purposes with a score of <20) with the first axis. Axes are thus selected in order that aspects of the subject's matrix can be visually represented because it is of value to determine which constructs are major in terms of accounting for more of the variance. However, the raw correlation matrix itself remains a major source of information.

In essence repertory grids are forms of sorting test. They differ from conventional sorting tests in that there are no standard sorting materials or categories, both can be supplied to or elicited from individual patients in terms of the area under investigation. Their other unique characteristic is that what is measured is the relationship between the sorting categories (concepts, ideas) for the subject and not the "correctness" of the sorts as such.

GRID I

One constant statement used by the patient whenever he discussed his acts of arson was that the important time for him when lighting fires was the moment between putting the match to the fire and the flames leaping up. When the fire had taken hold he was horrified by what he had done and would go quickly away.

This grid was designed to determine which was the most important; the moment of putting the match to the fire, the moment the flames were about to flare up, the blaze or the smell of the fire and to compare the feeling experienced by the patient with other emotion-evoking situations.

The constructs were all supplied in terms of the aims outlined above. The elements were adjectival descriptions of emotions as follows: Disturbing, Tearful, Shameful, Revengeful, Peaceful, Dangerous, Exhilarating, Angry, Guilty. The patient was presented with a construct such as "the smell of a wood fire burning" and asked to select the adjective that was most descriptive of the feeling aroused by the situation, the other adjectives then being ranked in order of appropriateness.

Results

The major axis "the moment before the fire gets under way" is quite unrelated to "the blaze of a fire" or "the smell of a wood fire burning" but involves the same sort of feeling as that ex-

Fig. 1. Constructs for Grid I plotted along the two main independent axes. Elements were adjectival descriptions of emotions.

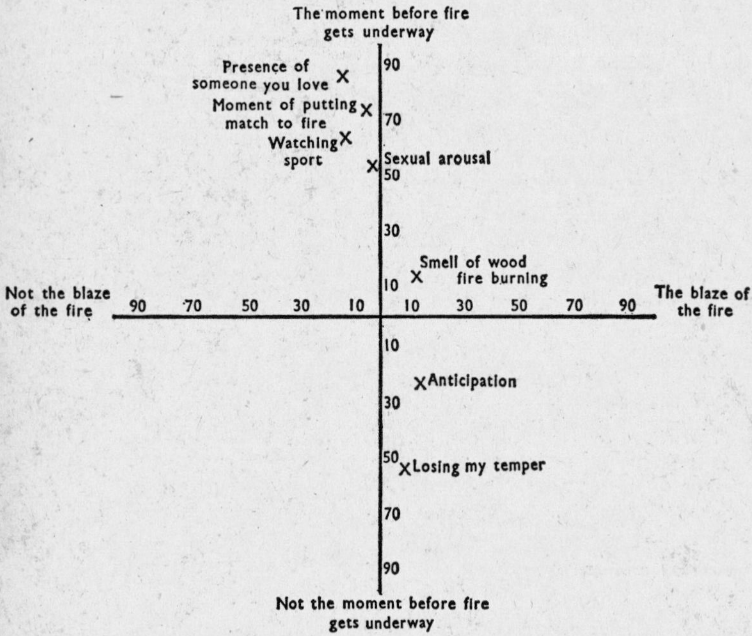

perienced when "putting the match to the fire" (rho = +0.89). The important moments in fire lighting appear to be, as the patient had stated, the short interval between putting the match to the fire and the appearance of the flames.

Figure 1 shows that nearly all the emotion-evoking situations used in the grid are significantly related to the feeling experienced when lighting a fire.

GRID II

The aims were (i) to attempt to find a construct which would be related to the feelings experienced while lighting a fire and to either "being sexually aroused" or "watching sport" and (ii) to provide a general description of the patient's personal construct system.

Eight constructs were elicited and ten supplied. The constructs were supplied on the basis that they (i) had been shown to be related to fire lighting in the first grid, (ii) were necessary for a comprehensive description of a person's construct system in the area of interpersonal relationships (e.g. the self and ideal self constructs) and (iii) might be expected to throw some light on the nature of the feeling experienced by the patient when he had just lit a fire, e.g. "creative" and "crave excitement." The construct "likely to commit arson" was used to see how the patient related this aspect of his act to his view of himself and the feelings experienced during the act.

The elements used were ten people known to and selected by the patient. Thus the patient was asked to select the person who was, for example, most "upright" in character and to rank in order the remaining people in terms of this construct down to the person who was least "upright."

Results

The main axes (Fig. 2) were "like I'd like to be in character" and "like watching sport." The ideal-self construct and "upright" were identical for the patient (rho = +1.0). It was quite arbitrary which construct was selected as the main axis along which the other constructs were to be plotted.

This grid can be regarded as a valid description of the patient's view of the world in so far as it tallies with what many might expect from someone who, like the patient, was brought up by strict, puritanical parents in an environment where ideas of sex and self-indulgence were punished and where duty and self-discipline were highly valued. Figure 2 is consistent with this background in showing "as I'd like to be in character," "upright," "decisive," "strict" and "like me in character" clustered at one

Fig. 2. Constructs for Grid II plotted along the two main independent axes. Elements were people known to the patient.

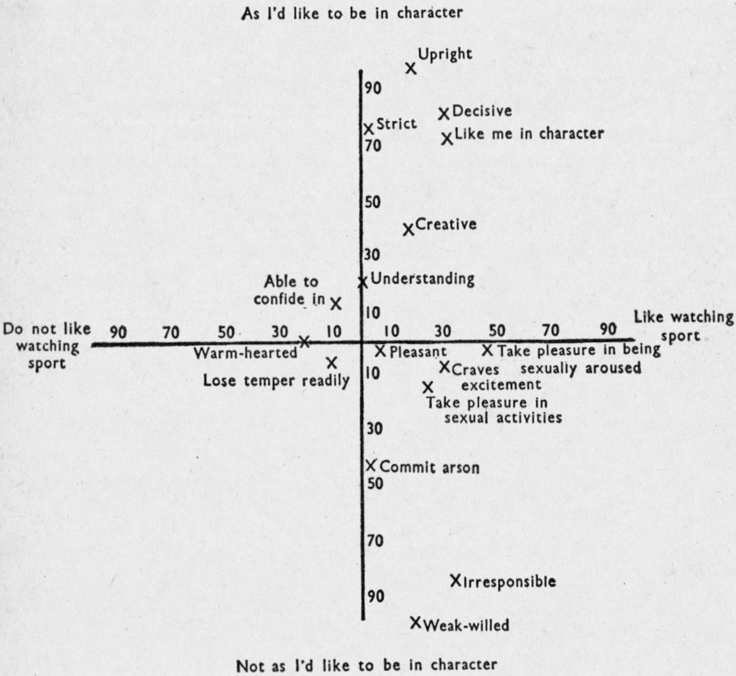

pole of the major axis and "as I'd *not* like to be," "weak-willed" and "irresponsible" clustered at the opposite pole.

An aim of this grid was to find a construct that would relate the feelings the patient experienced while lighting a fire to either those involved when sexually aroused or when watching sport. Figure 2 shows that the sex and sport constructs are significantly related to the fire construct (rho = +0.71 and +0.65) as well as to "crave excitement." The expectation that it would be possible to split these constructs so that only one remained related to fire lighting was not fulfilled if an analysis of Figure 2 alone is used. However, a grid based on a correlation matrix gives information on the relationship between all constructs with each other. An analysis of the self construct shows that the patient sees himself as someone who enjoys watching sport (rho = +0.60) but is indifferent to "pleasure in being sexually aroused" (rho = +0.05). Although the feelings he has watching sport, being sexually aroused and lighting a fire are related to *each other,* he only related feelings about fire and sport to *his view of himself.*

The fire-associated feeling is seen to be positively related to all good and desirable qualities as seen by this man but to have a negative correlation with "likely to commit arson." Also unpredicted was the finding of a significant negative correlation between the self and arson constructs. Grid III was constructed to explore *inter alia,* these two findings.

GRID III

This grid was designed to investigate whether feelings of hostility, revenge and power rather than sex are related by the patient to those experienced while lighting a fire.

All constructs were supplied and to vary the elements ten photographs of men were used.

Results

The two major axes are identical with those in Grid II. However, that "watching sport" emerged as the second axis was the result of its being the only construct that was not significantly correlated with the major axis it having, in fact, very little relation with any other construct in the grid.

The constructs polarize in a clear-cut way at the two poles of the ideal-self axis. People who enjoy having power and who believe others get the punishment they deserve are as the patient would like to be and as he sees himself as being, while those who take pleasure in being sexually aroused, commit arson and who are hostile and revengeful are as the patient would *not* like to be nor does he see himself thus. There is little discrepancy between his views of himself as he is and as he would like to be.

In general the same construct patterning recurs even now that different elements have again been used. Specifically, the feelings experienced while lighting a fire are once more highly correlated with the "good" pole of constructs and unrelated to sexual feelings and the significant negative correlation between the self and the sort of person who is likely to commit arson is again manifest. Subject to confirmation it seems to be the idea of power and not revenge nor hostility that is associated with fire-related feelings.

The only important change between Grids II and III is the reconstruing of "pleasure in being sexually aroused." Previously the psychiatric interviews were aimed at establishing whether or not the patient experienced sexual feelings during the fire lighting. Although the questioning was indirect, the patient was no doubt aware of the implications. Personal Construct Theory would account for this reconstruing of sex from being acceptable but unrelated to the self to being unacceptable and negatively related to the self by arguing that under questioning the patient was being forced to evaluate sexual feelings in relation to himself. In view of his puritanical upbringing it could be predicted that he would be forced to construe it as bad, which he did, at the same time "tightening" the related parts of his construct system. The end result of this reconstruction process is defined by constructs that are now significantly correlated with the "sex" construct, i.e. "like I'd like to be" −0.93; "the feelings I get when just having put a match to a fire" −0.96; "like me" −0.77; "hostile" +0.92; "likely to commit arson" +0.87.

In Fig. 3 one end of the scale shows that the man views himself as someone who enjoys power (+0.78), who believes people get the punishment they deserve (+0.95), who is as he would like to be (+0.92) and who relates all these ideas to the feelings experienced when lighting a fire. At the other pole are those who take pleasure in being sexually aroused, are hostile, seek revenge if they feel wronged and who, above all, are the sort of people who commit arson. This negative relationship between the self and arson constructs seemed particularly inconsistent in a man who "believes people get the punishment they deserve" and who has in fact confessed to the crime of arson. One highly speculative theory that would account for this inconsistency is to view this man as someone who is carrying on a crusade against those at the "like I'd *not* like to be" pole of his ideal-self construct. Not only does he believe in the cliché "people get the punishment they deserve" but he actively enjoys the power of punishing

Fig. 3. Constructs for Grid III plotted along the two main independent axes. Elements were ten photographs of men.

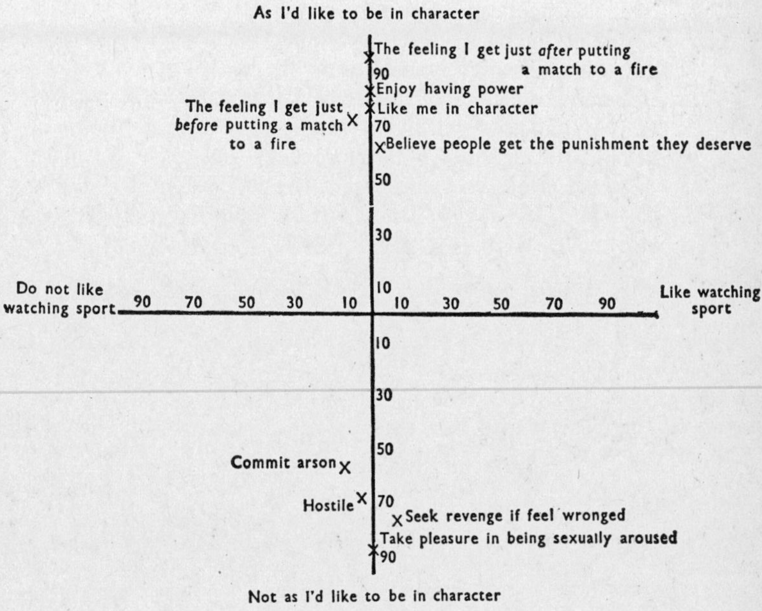

wrongdoers and sinners. In view of the very high relationship between all "good" qualities and the feelings he gets while putting a match to a fire, this act could be regarded as a symbolic purification of all those who have sinned. Clearly, such an act would not be regarded as wrong or criminal since he is meting out justice. Such an interpretation would only be of use if it were testable. It was therefore predicted in the next grid that the construct "people who punish wrongdoers" would be positively and significantly correlated with "like me," "upright" and the fire-related feelings, while "those who deserve punishment" would be positively and significantly correlated with "sinful," "irresponsible" and "pleasure in being sexually aroused." These predictions were at least consistent with the patient's history.

GRID IV

This grid was aimed at testing the hypotheses outlined above and at seeing how the patient related the construct "hostile" to his view of his wife.

The constructs were all supplied, some being selected because from previous analysis their meaning was regarded as relatively stable and their intercorrelations as predictable, viz.—"like I'd like to be" and "irresponsible" approximately −0.9 and "like I'd like to be" and "like me" approximately +0.9 and others supplied specifically to test the hypotheses. The same ten photographs of men were used as in Grid III.

Results

This is a one-axis grid (Fig. 4) as was Grid III with all constructs except "watching sport" being significantly related to "irresponsible." As predicted the correlation of "like I'd like to be" with "irresponsible" was −0.98 and with "like me" was +0.93.

The relationships of constructs with "those who deserve punishment" and "those who punish wrongdoers" are in line with the hypotheses.

Taking one line of thought to its limits we might regard this man as a crusader who sees himself as someone who is out to punish wrongdoers and his fire-lighting activities can be likened to symbolic acts of purification, conceptually he may be a "burner of heretics."

The patient still construes himself as non-hostile although the psychiatric interviews continued to be dominated by verbal expressions of hostility toward his wife. It was as if he found it necessary to provide a satisfactory explanation for his acts of arson. He had rejected the sexual connexion and was "trying out" the hostility idea, saying that he felt such hostility toward his wife that he lit a fire to provide an outlet for these feelings. The task he had presented himself with was to reconstrue "hostile"

Fig. 4. Constructs for Grid IV plotted along the two main independent axes. Elements were ten photographs of men.

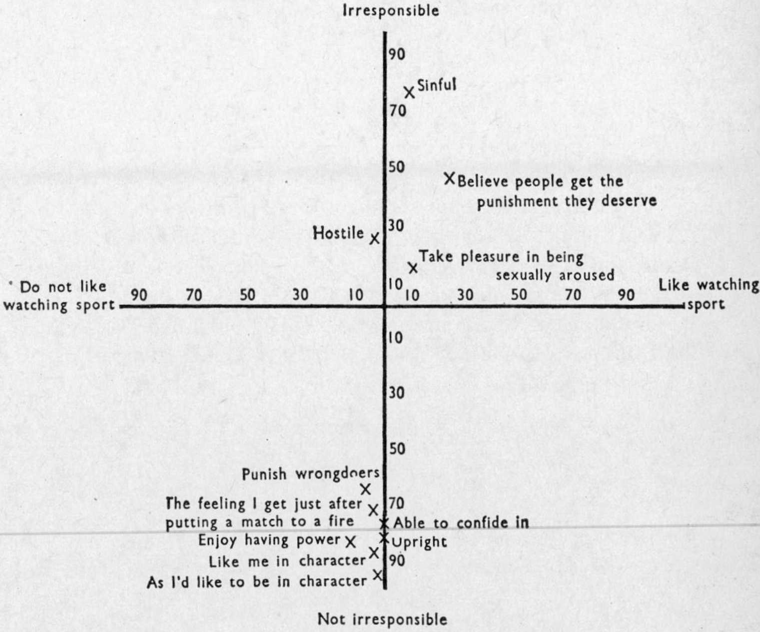

so that it was a desirable quality and thus could be related to "upright" people and so to himself.

GRID V

This grid was designed to elaborate the construct "sinful" in terms of immorality and femininity and to investigate whether further variation in elements would disrupt the construct patterning.

The elements consisted of ten photographs of women since one of the present aims was to analyse the relationship between sinfulness, femininity and immorality.

Results

The two independent axes (Fig. 5) are "like my wife in character" and "like my mother in character." Many of the previously obtained very high construct intercorrelations have been

Fig. 5. Constructs for Grid V plotted along the two main independent axes. Elements were ten photographs of women.

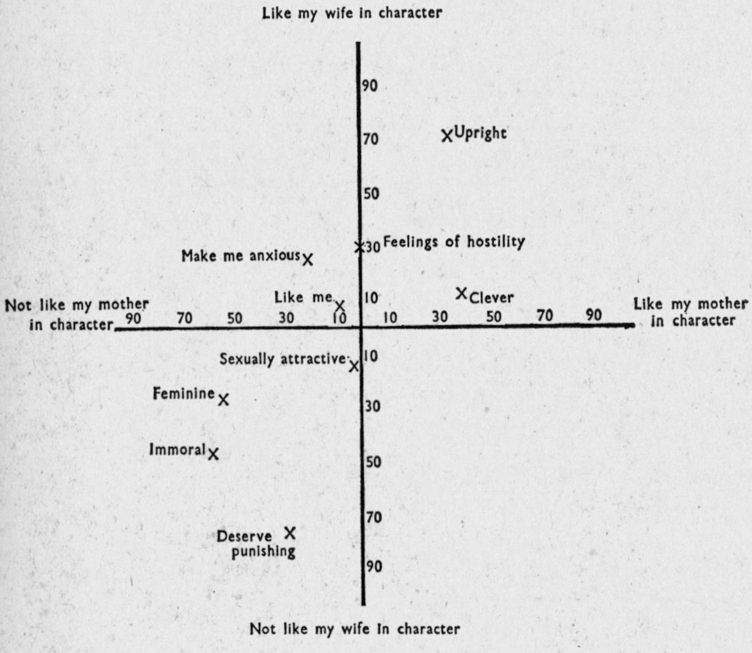

drastically reduced, particularly that between "like me" and "upright." The high correlations that are retained relate to his view of his wife who is "upright" (+0.88) and does *not* deserve punishing (0.88). There are two possible hypotheses to account for this breakdown of expected construct patterning. Either the patient has suffered a general loss of structure and is going through a crisis which makes him unable to construe what sort of person he is, or else the elements are outside the *range of convenience* of the construct "like me in character," i.e. the patient is unable to see any likeness in character between himself and the women in the photographs. If there were several elements outside the range of convenience of some constructs this would have the effect of lowering all correlations involving those constructs.

GRID VI

This final grid was designed to test whether the patient has experienced a genuine repatterning of his construct system or whether the constructs were outside the range of convenience of the elements. In order to enable direct comparison to be made the constructs were all supplied and the elements were the same ten people known to the patient used in Grid II.

Results

The major axis (Fig. 6) in relation to which the patient construes his environment and predicts events is "like I'd like to be in character" as it was in three of the previous grids and once again all other constructs are significantly correlated with it except "likely to be in the army."

A comparison with Grid II clearly shows that there has been no fundamental change in this man's construct system. The constructs are now more clearly polarized with the self, ideal self, fire-related feelings, "upright," feelings of hostility and power at the "good" pole and people who are immoral, sinful and who commit arson all being "deserving of punishment" at the "bad" pole. The one change of note being that people viewed as having feelings of hostility are now at the "good" pole. Such similarity between grids separated by 4 weeks and many psychotherapeutic sessions gives an indication of the stability or perhaps rigidity of this man's basic construct system. In view of this similarity it seemed justifiable to accept the loss of structure observed in Grid V as being due to the elements (female photographs) being outside the range of convenience of some of the constructs.

Fig. 6. Constructs for Grid VI plotted along the two main independent axes. Elements were ten people known to the patient.

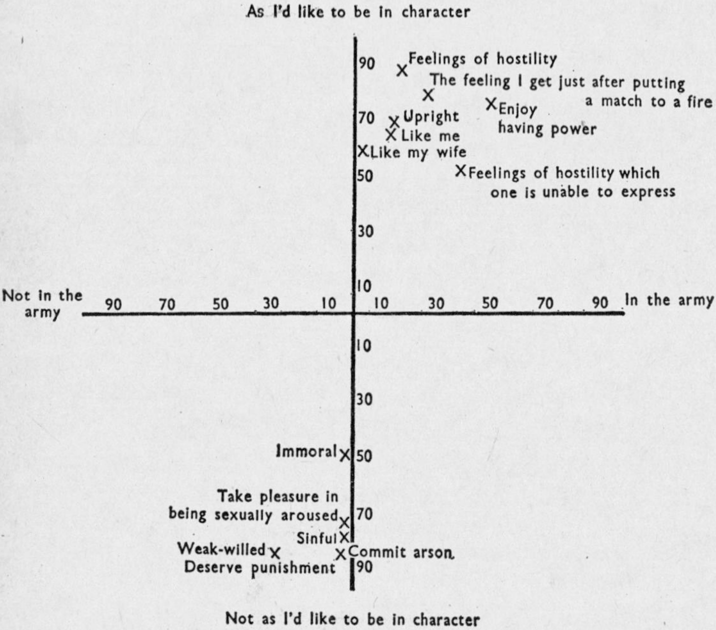

DISCUSSION

Validity

This series of repertory grids can be said to demonstrate the internal validity of the technique. That is, the presence of significant correlations is internal proof that the patient's grid behaviour is patterned and meaningful rather than random.

The use of people known to the patient as elements gave the technique content validity but the construct patterns are shown to be equivalent despite changes of element so that, providing the range of convenience rule is met, the photographs as elements could be said to give valid results.

The predictive validity of the technique can be tested by checking inferences from one grid to a succeeding grid (with psychotherapeutic manipulation as the intervening variable). Alternatively, views of the patient's clinical state and history can be translated into expected constant patterns and these checked by grid testing. The reported study suggests a degree of predictive validity in "grid to grid" terms.

Reliability

Detailed reliability studies on the method of repertory grid testing have yet to be reported. From this series it is possible to suggest the sort of reliabilities that may be expected. Constructs that were used in three or more grids are presented in Table 1.

TABLE 1

Showing Spearman rho's on Four Grids between the Construct "Like Me" and Those Listed

Constructs	Elements (people)	Elements (photographs)	Elements (photographs)	Elements (people)
Like me vs. Like I'd like to be	+0·88	+0·92	+0·93	+0·84
Like me vs. Enjoy power	—	+0·78	+0·89	+0·87
Like me vs. Upright	+0·88	—	+0·94	+1·00
Like me vs. Feelings re fire	+0·87	+0·88	+0·93	+0·89
Like me vs. Pleasure in being sexually aroused	+0·05	−0·77	−0·39	−0·39
Like me vs. Likely to commit arson	−0·59	−0·75	—	−0·90

The time interval between the first and fourth grids was about one month. The correlations from Grid V with "women" elements have not been quoted because they are regarded as being invalid due to the elements being outside the range of convenience of the constructs.

The stability of the relationship of the self construct with the first four constructs is clearly demonstrated. It is of interest to note the tendency for the negative relationship between the self and arson constructs to increase over time to the point where his view of himself approaches the direct opposite of the sort of person who commits arson. The changes that occurred between the self and sex constructs have been discussed earlier.

Uses of the Technique

This study merely attempts to illustrate a way in which the technique can be used in the study of the single case. There would seem to be considerable scope for its development as a device for testing hypotheses arising out of psychiatric enquiry.

Apart from its function as an aid to psychotherapeutic enquiry with the individual patient, it seems possible that certain generalizations can in time be derived which will enable indices for, say, prognosis to be developed. An example of a possible prognostic measure is the relationship between the "self" and constructs describing a major symptom of the patient. Grids given to neurotic patients very often have a zero or negative correlation between these two constructs and there is an indication that the correlation tends in a positive direction as the patient's condition improves. Following this line of thought this patient who has a correlation of –0.90 between the sort of person he thinks he is and the sort of person who commits arson, could be expected to commit that crime again should the right environmental ingredients present themselves, if for no other reason than that he is not in his view "committing arson."

REFERENCES

BANNISTER, D. (1962). Personal construct theory: A summary and experimental paradigm. *Acta Psychol. 20*, 104–120.

BANNISTER, D. (1963). The genesis of schizophrenic thought disorder: A serial invalidation hypothesis. *Brit. J. Psychiat. 109*, 680–686.

KELLY, G. A. (1955). *The Psychology of Personal Constructs,* vols. 1 and 2. New York: Norton.

LEWIS, N. D. C. & YARNELL, H. (1951). Pathological firesetting. *J. nerv. ment. Dis. 82.*

MARC, M. (1833). Consideration Medico-Legàle sur la Monomanie particulièrement sur la Monomanie Incendaire. *Ann. Hyg. publ. Paris, 10,* 367.

PILGRIM, C. W. (1884). Pyromania (so-called) with report of a case. *Amer. J. Insan. 41,* 457.

PRITCHARD, J. C. (1822). *A Treatise on Diseases of the Nervous System,* vol. I. London.

6

An Experimental Investigation of Disordered Motor Expression in a Catatonic Schizophrenic Patient*

H. R. BEECH and R. C. PARBOOSINGH

Five experiments were conducted in an attempt to explain the mechanisms underlying disordered motor expression in a catatonic schizophrenic patient. Two main conclusions were suggested by the experimental findings. First, that the motor symptoms were subject to disinhibition by an extraneous stimulus, and secondly that the lack of verbal responsiveness was related to defective verbal-motor output rather than to disordered sensory input.

INTRODUCTION

Although mannerisms and gesticulations are a common feature of schizophrenic disorders it would appear that relatively little attention has been paid by psychiatrists and psychologists to a systematic experimental investigation and explanation of such manifestations. The work reported here represents an attempt to establish some degree of experimental control over the mannerisms manifested by a female patient suffering from catatonic schizophrenia. Although the investigation could not be carried through to a satisfactory conclusion it seemed to the authors that certain generalizations could be made about the disordered motor expression in this patient which might hold for others suffering from the same kind of illness. Such generalizations might form the basis of an adequate theoretical account of mannerisms of

* Reprinted from the *British Journal of Social and Clinical Psychology,* 1962, Vol. I, pp. 222–227, by permission of the authors and the publisher.

this type, and provide some notions as to the mechanisms underlying such disorders.

The patient, an unmarried woman aged forty-six, suffered her first recorded mental illness three years prior to her present attack, and during this period was hospitalized for seven months with a diagnosis of catatonic schizophrenia. The same diagnosis was made during her most recent illness.

At the time of her second attack, when the investigation reported here was carried out, the patient was described as tense, anxious, aggressive, incoherent in speech, and labile in mood. Her behaviour alternated between sobbing, giggling, and vacantly staring, and gesticulations were marked and frequently observed.

It was decided to investigate the nature of the peculiar gesticulations, which included rubbing the hands, tapping the head or other parts of the body, making clicking sounds with her tongue, bowing, and tapping nearby objects. One explanation was immediately suggested by a consideration of her history, namely that in trying to communicate with her deaf sister a variety of motor movements had been useful, and that these movements were perpetuated in her present illness as a form of communication with her present hospital environment. Such an explanation would be in accord with the generally held view that such movements ". . . have a definite psychological meaning, the symbolic significance in each case being peculiar to the individual and determined by his complexes or other affective experiences," Noyes (1953).

Further support for this kind of explanation came from our first period of uncontrolled observation where it became clear that the patient was able to respond verbally to simple questions when *not* manifesting motor activity; during an "activity" phase, however, no verbal responses could be elicited. Such observations strongly suggested that the motor actions were a substitute for verbal communication.

It might also be argued that two other observations would be consistent with this explanation:

(*a*) When the same question is asked repeatedly by the investigator, the motor actions should be relatively consistent.

(*b*) When different questions are asked by the experimenter, the motor actions should vary according to the question.

EXPERIMENT I

Accordingly an attempt was made to code the motor expressions exhibited by the patient and these "responses" were noted whenever simple questions were asked. The gestures used by the patient were too numerous and too quickly made to make recording reliable, but the outcome strongly suggested that no relationships existed between the questions asked and the subsequent gesticulations made by the patient. In other words, the same question was capable of eliciting a variety of different motor "responses," and different questions seemed capable of eliciting the same motor "response" by the patient.

It has already been mentioned that the patient's behaviour was characterized by two distinct phases; in one phase (hereafter called "activity") gesticulations were present but verbal responses were absent, while in the other phase (hereafter called "inactivity") verbal responses could be elicited and gesticulations were absent. It therefore seemed appropriate to examine the possibility of interrupting the "activity" phase in some way in order to ascertain whether or not verbal responses could be obtained under such conditions.

EXPERIMENT II

Six simple questions were prepared and each question was presented twice under each of three experimental conditions in balanced order. The three conditions were as follows:

A. During "inactivity" (i.e. when no gesticulations were present).
B. During "activity" (i.e. when the patient was gesticulating).
C. During "activity" with distraction (i.e. during an on-going "activity" phase a buzzer was sounded).

Under condition C an attempt was made to reduce possible habituation to the distracting stimulus by presenting the three possible combinations of one long and two short "buzzes" in random order.

The procedure of presenting questions under these three conditions was carried out on two different days, the repetition of the procedure on the second day being necessary to ensure the reliability of our observations. The results, as shown in Table 1 indicate a high degree of consistency in the patient's behaviour

TABLE 1

Number of Correct Responses Given under the three Experimental Conditions A, B, and C

	A	B	C
Day 1	12	5	11
Day 2	10	1	10

Analysis of variance F ratios

Day 1: $F = 6{\cdot}08$, $p > 0{\cdot}01$
t (Condition B × Condition C) = 3·35, $p = 0{\cdot}05$
Day 2: $F = 11{\cdot}57$, $p > 0{\cdot}01$
t (Condition B × Condition C) = 5·72, $p = 0{\cdot}01$

in spite of her mood changing from elation to aggression and the fact that on the first occasion she had taken 3 grains of sodium amytal while on the second she had received no drugs.

In this experiment scoring was concerned with correct verbal responses to the questions asked, and reference to Table 1 indicates that on both occasions of testing the patient produced about as many correct verbal responses under conditions of distraction as under "inactivity" conditions. On the other hand, when tested under "activity" conditions without distraction the patient produced only six correct verbal responses to the twenty-four questions asked on the two test sessions.

It should be noted that the distraction conditions not only produced the modifications in verbal responsiveness referred to above, but also resulted in cessation of gesticulatory behaviour.

The difference between scores obtained on conditions A and C do not differ significantly, while the differences between conditions B and C, and between conditions A and B, do achieve an acceptable level of statistical significance.

These results indicate that the phenomenon has been brought under some degree of experimental control, and that conditions have been provided under which it is possible to "normalize" the patient's verbal behaviour and terminate an "activity" phase.

EXPERIMENT III

A second stage of the investigation was then conducted in which we tried to establish whether the diminished ability to produce adequate verbalization during an activity phase was due to defect in sensory input or verbal-motor output. The technique chosen for this was to ask questions during "activity" periods and elicit responses, without repeating the questions, during "inactivity" phases. For example, a question such as "Do you prefer peaches or bananas?" was asked during an "activity" period, and when this phase was terminated the examiner simply asked, "Which do you prefer?"

Unfortunately the patient would not respond to this forced-choice test other than by citing personal preferences *in the appropriate category;* for example, in response to the sample question given above, she simply named her favourite fruit. The tendency for the patient to respond to these questions by producing a *correct category* answer was highly significant ($p = 0.0002$), and therefore cannot be accounted for by chance. These results already suggested that during "activity" the patient was capable of receiving and recording impressions, but was unable to produce adequate verbal responses until she went into an "inactivity" phase. However, in order to obtain more clear-cut evidence it was decided to simplify the nature of the stimuli and to present them tactually and visually as well as in the auditory modality. The patient's task was to recognize, when in an "inactive" period, the stimulus which had been presented during an "active" phase.

Our fourth experiment was therefore directed at attempting to confirm the results of Experiment III, and to examine the possibility that the "activity" phase did not interfere with sensory input in any modality but operated so as to restrict verbal motor output.

EXPERIMENT IV

In the case of testing our hypothesis for the visual modality, six differently coloured cards were employed, one of which was presented during an "active" phase. When the patient moved into a period of "inactivity" she was asked to recognize the appropriate stimulus colour from a choice of three coloured cards.

Altogether nine test trials were completed, and in eight of these the patient successfully identified the correct stimulus square. This score achieves a high level of significance ($p = 0.0004$) and is well beyond the score which would be expected by chance alone.

Essentially the same task was employed for auditory presentation. Here, the name of one of six different colours was spoken by the experimenter during an "activity" period and the patient was asked to name this colour from a choice of three colour names given during an "inactive" phase. Out of nine test trials conducted in this way the patient gave five correct responses. Although the score was somewhat lower than that obtained on visual presentation it was nevertheless much greater than chance expectancy ($p = 0.006$).

The tactual recognition procedure was unfortunately spoiled by an error in administration and the results could not be evaluated.

In the case of both auditory and visual tests in Experiment IV our results support our hypothesis that the lack of verbal responsiveness during an "inactivity" phase is *not* due to defective sensory input. At least on the simple tasks employed by us it would seem that the most reasonable explanation is one which postulates some blocking or inhibition of verbal-motor output. The differential scores obtained by the patient on visual and auditory modality tests might be accounted for in terms of differences in memory ability under the two conditions of testing.

EXPERIMENT V

In order to obtain further evidence concerning the patient's responsiveness during "activity" and "inactivity" phases an experiment was carried out in which her reactions to simple commands were observed. Such commands (e.g. "Stand up," "Shut the door") were spoken during an "activity" phase, each of the ten commands given being repeated six times in random order.

It was found that the patient was immediately able to carry out all these instructions without waiting for an "inactivity" phase, so that the results do not support the general position adopted before this experiment was conducted. However, three factors might be usefully considered in evaluating the apparent discrepancy between earlier experiments in which the patient did not respond to auditory stimuli during an "activity" period, and Experiment V where she responded immediately under these conditions.

First, at the time of the last experiment the patient had commenced a course of E.C.T., and it could be argued that this variable might have significantly affected the consistent trend of results previously obtained. Secondly, perhaps as a result of the E.C.T., it had become increasingly difficult to judge whether or not the patient actually was in an "activity" or an "inactivity" phase, and mistakes in the time of administration of the auditory stimulus could have been made.

A third point concerning the discrepancy might be in terms of the mechanisms affected by the patient's disorder. In the first four experiments the subject had been required to produce *verbal* responses during "activity," while in the last experiment all the commands given required a purely *motor* response. The apparent discrepancy might therefore be a function of the mode of response required, and one would need to argue that while verbal-motor responsiveness is inhibited during "activity" no such impediment exists in other aspects of motor responsiveness.

At this stage of the investigation it was decided to abandon the project in view of the patient's very rapid return to normality, and it was therefore not possible to decide which of the three points raised, or which combinations of those factors, were responsible for the apparent discrepancy.

DISCUSSION

The initial observations made, namely, that the activity–non-activity behaviour appeared to be fairly regular and cyclic, and that verbal responses could be elicited in one phase but not in the other, suggest that some kind of inhibitory potential is built up from time to time which prevents adequate verbalization. One might ask whether, in this case, the movements represent the patient's attempt at self-disinhibition, or some kind of spontaneous and involuntary change in the direction of flow of cerebral impulses from motor-speech to purely motor functions.

It seems unreasonable to say that the motor movements made by the patient are themselves disinhibitors as the buzzer results in the cessation of such movements and immediately restores verbal communication. A more plausible account would appear to be that the motor activity represents some spontaneous, involuntary, and cyclic switching of impulses or innervation as a result of blocking in verbal-motor output. In other words, it may be possible to conceive of the development of an active preventative process in verbal-motor output "channels" leading to the spontaneous discharge of energy via other purely motor "channels." Under ordinary circumstances during an "activity" period the accumulated inhibition in the former is allowed to dissipate; under other circumstances (e.g. when a strong extraneous stimulus is presented) the verbal-motor channel might be subject to disinhibition, or alternatively the purely motor channel might be inhibited thus releasing the verbal-motor channel for use.

Two further assumptions might also be made. First, that once one of the "channels" is in use such usage is continued in a limited perseverative way; secondly, that an active "blocking" process rapidly develops in any "channel" in current use. These assumptions enable us to account for the fluctuating cyclic nature of the dysfunction.

It would, of course, be necessary to decide by experiment whether the extraneous stimulus operates so as to disinhibit the channel in use. Once in use, as indicated above, the channel in use reciprocally inhibits other channels.

REFERENCE

NOYES, P. N. (1953). *Modern Clinical Psychiatry*. London: W. B. Saunders Co.

7

An Investigation of an Abnormality of Cognitive Function in a Cooperative Young Psychotic: An Example of the Application of Experimental Method to the Single Case*

M. B. SHAPIRO and E. H. NELSON

THE SINGLE CASE IN EXPERIMENTAL PSYCHIATRY

It has been argued elsewhere (*8, 9, 11*) that the systematic objective investigation of a single abnormality in a single case should lead to findings which are relevant to the general function of the individual concerned and which can be generalised to many other individuals. The first attempt to check this viewpoint is reported in the papers quoted above. The investigation reported in these papers began with the experimental investigation of an apparent anomaly of perceptual function in a psychiatric patient. As a result, some of the laws determining the appearance of the anomaly were established. Further investigation showed that the anomaly appeared most frequently amongst brain damaged patients. An explanation was then formulated, accounting for the facts that the anomaly obeyed these particular laws and appeared most frequently in brain damaged patients. This explanation, which had implications for the general adjustment of brain damaged patients, also permitted precise deductions. One of these deductions was the conditions which would make a normal per-

* Reprinted from the *Journal of Clinical Psychology,* Oct. 1955, Vol. XI, No. 4, pp. 344–351, by permission of the authors and the publisher.

son also show the perceptual anomaly and do so according to the same laws. Experiment confirmed these deductions.

It might be argued that the apparently successful outcome of this investigation was partly due to chance and partly due to the fact that we were dealing with an anomaly which was related to brain damage. It was, therefore, necessary to start another investigation of this type in a patient who was suffering from a functional disorder. This paper reports such an investigation.

Before reporting this investigation it is necessary to deal briefly with the underlying theoretical conceptions. The first of these is that the individual's total behavior and experience is a function of the interaction of various aspects of psycho-physiological function. The experimental investigation of the causes of any single abnormality of psychological function may, therefore, lead to an improved understanding of the patient's abnormality as a whole. The second conception is that the understanding of the psychological dysfunction of any single patient may be relevant to the understanding of the disorders of many other patients. It should be stated at this point that any function is regarded as psychological if the subject reports that conscious experience has been in any way involved.

These conceptions have to be made explicit because many psychologists and psychiatrists appear to work on the unproven assumption that the precise investigation of any single aspect of function in a single case *must* result in unique findings, findings which will be incapable of generalization, either to other aspects of the individual's function, or to the same function in other people. This assumption has done much to paralyse effective experimental work in clinical psychology.

The effectiveness of an investigation of a single aspect of function in a single case depends, however, on the rigour with which it is carried out. To quote from a previous paper (*9*): "By rigour is meant, first of all, that no experiment is ever conducted unless a formulated explanatory hypothesis is being tested. Secondly, no hypothesis is ever considered unless testable deductions can be made from it. Such deductions must result in experiments in which the phenomenon concerned varies its appearance in a manner which confirms or contradicts the hypothesis. Such an approach would, of course, become an empty drill, if the hypotheses which are developed are not explanatory and capable of wider application beyond the immediate limits of the point of the investigation."

THE INITIAL OBSERVATION

The initial observation which started the investigation reported in this paper was the fact that a 22 year old male psychiatric patient, who had obtained well above average scores on cognitive tests such as the Wechsler, was unable to understand simple material when he read it aloud. The Wechsler-Bellevue scores are given below:

FULL SCALE I. Q. 118

Verbal Scale I. Q. 120		*Performance Scale I. Q. 113*	
Comprehension	13	Picture Arrangement	11
Digit Span	11	Picture Completion	11
Arithmetic	10	Block Design	15
Similarities	13	Object Assembly	14
Vocabulary	15	Digit Symbol	9

PSYCHIATRIC SUMMARY OF THE SUBJECT

The patient had his first breakdown at the age of 20 while he was studying for his degree as a resident student of a university. This breakdown was preceded by a period of inability to concentrate on his studies, and of apparent "withdrawal" from his fellow students, teachers and relatives. Under psychiatric observation he was, in addition, reported to have rapid variations in mood, "significant thoughts," suspiciousness and panics. He was given 40 insulin comas, and made an apparent recovery. After spending some months hitch-hiking and working his way around a country abroad he returned to his university, and recommenced his studies in the autumn term. He felt very well until December of that year when he again found difficulty with his concentration, with attendant anxiety about his mental state. He finally became "depressed" and "perplexed" and was given another 40 insulin comas and 6 E. C. T. with considerable improvement. It was at this phase that he was seen by our psychological department. In the testing situation he appeared to be an extremely cooperative, pleasant, sensible and persistent person.

He is reported to have been a happy child but shy, easily frightened and crying easily. No other abnormal traits are reported. At school he was a good average scholar, active socially and good at games. He passed school certificate but failed higher schools. On leaving school he went into the Army for two years and obtained a commission. His father is a successful professional worker, and the home environment is apparently kindly and cultured. He is reported to have shown no interest in sex and not to have had either homo- or heterosexual experiences. The patient had complained that he found it difficult to read books and in order to check this complaint the reading comprehension tests were given.

OBJECTIVE CONFIRMATION OF THE COMPLAINT

In order to confirm the patient's complaint, two tests were given: the Schonell Prose Reading Test "My Dog" and the Schonell Silent Reading Test A (7).

Schonell Prose Reading Test "My Dog" (7). In this test the subject has to read aloud a simple story. Three scores are recorded: the number of mistakes in actual reading, the time taken to read the passage, and the number of standard questions on the content of the story which can be answered correctly.

RESULTS:

(a) *Reading Mistakes.* <9.5 years (the ceiling of this test is at 9.5 years).
(b) *Reading Speed.* Between 8.5 years and 9.5 years (the ceiling is at 9.5 years).
(c) *Answering Oral Questions on the Test.* Four out of 15 were answered correctly, giving a reading age of less than 6 years.

It seemed from these results that the patient could make correct oral responses to print, but did so slowly and with almost no comprehension of what he had read. In the light of his full scale Wechsler score and his school record, this lack of comprehension was regarded as being abnormal and as confirming the patient's claim that he had only been able to read through one book in whole of his life. It was decided to make the apparent abnormality of performance on this reading test the starting point of the investigation.

Schonell Silent Reading Test A (*7*). In this test the subject is left to read a number of passages to himself. Each passage is followed by printed questions which the patient has to answer in writing. The correctness of the subject's answers to these questions gives a measure of the subject's comprehension of what he has read. Two scores are derived: accuracy and speed. On the first he broke the ceiling of the test which goes up to 13½ year level. On the second he obtained a score between 10 and 11 years.

PRELIMINARY HYPOTHESES

Seven explanatory hypotheses were set up in the early stages of the investigation. For the sake of brevity of exposition they will be stated at the outset, though in fact they were formulated at different times. It should be noted that these hypotheses were not mutually exclusive. The hypotheses were:

(i) The patient had a specific reading defect.
(ii) The patient fatigued very quickly.
(iii) He had difficulty in attaching meaning to words.
(iv) The patient had a reading comprehension difficulty which was characteristic of some schizophrenics.
(v) The patient was extremely slow in reading comprehension.
(vi) "My Dog" is psychologically an inappropriate test for adults. It could be argued that reading simple material aloud was both an unaccustomed and embarrassing task for adults.

TESTING THE HYPOTHESES OF A SPECIFIC READING DEFECT AND FATIGUABILITY

A number of actions were taken to investigate these two hypotheses:

1. The history of the patient was investigated. This revealed that the patient had never been backward in reading. He claimed, however, that he had had as a child a tendency to read from right to left, to make reversals such as "on" for "no." His cultured family had teased him, he said, for his so-called backwardness.
2. His present reading habits were checked. No clear-cut abnormalities could be observed such as eye-voice lag, or reading words singly. The only thing which was clearly confirmed was his claimed inability to take in what he read.
3. In order to establish the limit of his comprehension in silent reading as against reading aloud, he was given the Schornell Silent Reading Test B. This test has a ceiling of 15 years.

At the same time the hypothesis of easy fatiguability was checked by preceding the Reading test with the first two subtests of the Wechsler Verbal Scale and then following the reading test immediately with the rest of the Wechsler test. The Wechsler test results were required anyway, as it was necessary to check his present intellectual level. The patient appeared to be as efficient in the latter part of the Wechsler as in the early part. Grossly abnormal fatiguability was not observable here.

On the Silent Reading test he obtained a reading age of 12 years, answering 28 out of the 42 questions in the test correctly. He did not finish the test in the time limit of 15 minutes.

4. To ensure that there was not some actual disability which prevented the patient from finishing the Schonell Silent Reading Test B, and to check the hypothesis of slowness of reading comprehension, the patient was given the test to complete in his own time on the following day. This he did, and he obtained the maximum reading age of 15 years 2 months on the test. For the purposes of this investigation the hypothesis of a specific reading defect was dropped therefore at this stage.

CHECKING THE INAPPROPRIATENESS OF "MY DOG" AS A TEST FOR ADULTS

Here again a number of things were done.

1. The patient was given Burt's "King of the Golden River" (*1*). This test is similar to "My Dog" in that it consists of relatively

simple material which is read aloud and the subject is subsequently tested for comprehension by questions. This test was given to see if there was anything peculiar to the content or the conditions of the administration of "My Dog." The patient in fact obtained a reading age of 7 to 8 years on Burt's test, which was again far below what one would expect from the patient's intelligence level and record.

2. In order to check the standardization and the psychological appropriateness of the reading tests used so far, three of them were given to a sample of normal controls who were like the patient in social status and intellectual level. Most of them were Psychology graduates working in the department. The results were:

(i) *My Dog*. Nine subjects were tested. The range of scores was from 6 to 15 out of 15 questions answered correctly. The mean reading age was 8.5–9 years. Some of the controls obtained scores nearly as bad as that of our subject. The raw data have unfortunately been lost.

(ii) *King of the Golden River*.

Frequency	*Reading Age*	*No. Correct Answers*
5	9–10 years	9–11
1	11–12	12–13
1	12–13	13–14
2	13–14	14–16
Patient	7–8	5

Five of our controls obtained a score well below the ceiling of the test and only slightly superior to that of the patient. Only two of the controls just reached the ceiling of the test.

(iii) *Schonell Form B* (*Silent Reading Comprehension*). All nine subjects obtained the maximum score of 15 years 2 months for men and of 15 years for women within the time limit of 15 minutes.

Two conclusions emerge from these results. The first is that the controls found no difficulty with the silent reading situation as measured by Schonell Form B. Thus our patient's slowness of reading comprehension is confirmed.

The second conclusion is that our adult controls found it relatively difficult to comprehend simple material when they themselves read it aloud and that therefore the patient's difficulty in this test is not definitely abnormal. On the other hand we are not in a position to say that the patient showed no abnormality in this test for his score is still worse than any of the controls and the number of controls is too small to decide on the significance of this observation.

THE RELATION OF COMPREHENSION WHILE READING ALOUD TO SCHIZOPHRENIA

To check this relation "My Dog" was given to two schizophrenic patients of well above average intelligence, whose diagnoses were unequivocal.

Diagnosis	*Reading Age*	*Time Taken*	*No. Correct*	*C. A.*
Hebephrenic	6	50″	6	19
Paranoid schiz.	6	60″	6	24
Our patient	less than 6	86″ approx.	4	22

These results lie between our patient's and that of the control groups. Again, we have insufficient data to indicate the degree of abnormality of these findings.

RECAPITULATION AND REFORMULATION

Four main findings emerged from the data so far gathered:

1. There was a contraindication of the existence of a specific reading defect in the patient.
2. There was some evidence that the patient was not abnormally prone to fatigue in cognitive function.
3. There were good grounds for believing that the patient was relatively slow in the comprehension of printed matter.
4. There was clear evidence that the comprehension of simple material whilst reading it aloud is difficult for some normal adults. (At least they cannot do it better than children.)

The last of these results appeared to rob us of the apparently dramatic and clear cut abnormality which we seemed to have at the outset of the investigation. The disappearance of this abnormality was not, however, complete. Our patient was consistently worse than the controls in the reading tests, and the schizophrenics in turn were worse than the normals on "My Dog," though doing better than our patient. Our numbers were too small and our sampling too restricted to make an accurate estimate of the degree of abnormality of this finding. We were therefore not in a position to decide with any confidence for or against the existence in our patient of an abnormality, in the strict sense of the term, of reading comprehension as measured by "My Dog."

Two possible alternatives emerged from the situation: either to collect a considerable amount of control data on "My Dog" which would give us a reliable measure of the patient's degree of abnormality in this task, or to put forward an explanation of all the available results which could be tested by an adequately stndardized test. It was decided to do the second, if possible, as it was the less time consuming procedure.

A GENERAL EXPLANATION AND ITS VALIDATION

Further consideration of the results obtained suggested an explanation. This was that our patient was abnormally slow in any kind of cognitive function. This was indicated by his relative slowness in the silent reading comprehension test, a function which is known to be quite highly correlated with other types of cognitive tests. Our normal controls all exceeded the maximum score on this test. Slowness of cognition could also account for the patient's difficulty in comprehending what he had read aloud. If the patient's rate of responding verbally to print were relatively fast (as it was) then his rate of comprehension could not keep pace with rate of reading aloud. Fortunately an appropriately standardized and validated test was available to check the theory of the patient's cognitive slowness (*3, 4*). In fact its existence brought the hypothesis readily to mind. This test was Furneaux's speed and level test of inductive reasoning, which is based on Thurstone's letter series test.

Each item in this test is made up of a series of letters. Each series has a definite pattern of relationships. The subject has to work out the pattern and then complete the series. A simple example would be the AXAYBXBYCXC. The subject has to fill in the one letter indicated by the dot.

In the level test the subject is instructed to take as long with each item as he desires and only to respond with the answer when fully satisfied that it is correct. He is then given six practice items. When this practice is completed the subject goes on to the main part of the level test. This consists of three independent series of items. Each series consists of 7 items, each of which is on a separate card. The items of each series are graded in difficulty level from that passed by 80% of the normal population to that passed by 5%, and the graduation in each series is of the same order. Thus each individual has three opportunities to show the level he can reach.

The speed test is always given after the level test so that differences in learning and practice effects can be reduced. All the items of the speed test can be passed by 80% of the normal population. The subject is required to work as quickly as possible, to answer each item in turn without omitting any items. To facilitate scoring he is asked to make a circle around the last item completed whenever the examiner taps his pencil. This is done every 20 seconds. The essential virtue of the construction of the speed test lies in the fact that only the items which a subject does correctly are scored. The speed test therefore gives a measure of a subject's speed of successful function, and is not complicated by the time he spent on incorrectly completed items.

The results of the test were quite clear. The patient obtained a score of +.57 sigma on the level test. The standardization data were obtained from university undergraduates. On the speed test he obtained a score of −1.5 sigma. The discrepancy of 2.07 sigma between speed and level was extremely unusual. In Furneaux's control data there are 172 students who obtained a score between +.5 and +.6 sigma (this information was given in a private communication and is about to be published). Of these only three obtained a discrepancy of two sigma or more. The hypothesis that our patient was abnormally slow in cognitive function was confirmed.

To check on whether this abnormal discrepancy was a general

function of mental disorder, the speed and level tests were given to four diagnosed schizophrenics:

Patient	*Level**	*Speed**	*Level-Speed Discrepancy**
1	+0.86	−1.66	−2.52
2	+0.86	−3.1	−3.96
3	+1.85	+2.0	+0.15
4	+0.16	−2.56	−3.72

* All results are given in terms of standard deviations of the normal student sample.

Of these patients only No. 3, the one without a discrepancy, was rediagnosed before discharge. The new diagnosis was that of anxiety neurosis. According to Furneaux's data the remaining three discrepancies were at least as abnormal as that given by our patient. We thus appear to be dealing with an abnormality characteristic of at least some schizophrenics.

To check the link of this finding with slowness of reading, one more test was given. The patient was asked to read a story in a magazine. Fifteen questions were prepared to test the subject's comprehension. Our patient took 10½ minutes to read the story, silently to himself, and answered 14 out of 15 questions correctly. Eight normal controls ranged from 2½ to 7 minutes in reading the story and none answered fewer than 14 out of 15 questions correctly. All subjects were asked to read in their own time. It would seem, therefore, that the patient suffered from a general slowness of intellectual function and the reading difficulty may well be related to this slowness.

TESTING THE GENERALITY OF THE FINDING

It now remained for us to confirm the generality of the finding that some schizophrenics, while suffering little or no impairment of level of cognitive function, would be abnormally slow in carrying out such function. This investigation was carried out by Ogilvie (*6*).

He gave the Nufferno level and speed tests to 22 patients. The selection of patients was governed by the aim of making them as like our original patient as possible. Their average age was 24 years with a range from 18 to 36 years. They were all considered to be of above average intelligence in the opinion of their psychiatrists and at the time of testing were considered to be schizophrenic. They were all fully cooperative in the testing situation. The short form of the Nufferno Level Test and the interrupted form of the speed test described above were used. The results were compared, as before, with the data previously gathered from the university students.

The results were fully in line with expectation. The mean time per item successfuly completed by the patients was 16.5 seconds. The mean time taken by the university students was 6.9 seconds. The difference gave a "t" of 11.3 which was significant well beyond the .001 level of confidence. On the level tests, the mean score for the patients was lower than that of the students but the difference did not reach statistical significance.

The clear cut character of the results is further indicated when the patient's raw scores were transformed into standard scores on the basis of the student data. This enabled Ogilvie to compare the performance of each patient with that of the student controls, on each of the tests. In every case but two, the patients did relatively better on the level test than they did on the speed test. The generality of this finding was further confirmed by Eysenck in a parallel study (*2*), who reports results of giving the speed and level tests to non-university normals, neurotics and psychotics. He found that there was no difference between the three groups in the level of problem solving ability. The psychotics, however, were significantly slower than the other two groups. The normals and neurotics did not differ significantly in speed.

CONCLUSIONS

First, we have the incidental but useful finding that, compared with nine year old children, adults find it difficult to comprehend simple material which they read aloud. Whatever may be the cause of this difficulty, it argues for the need for considerable caution in the interpretation of an adult's score on a test which has been standardized on children.

Second, we have a finding of general importance. This finding directs attention to a form of impairment which tends to be ignored: a lowering of speed of cognitive function independently of level. Current concepts of deterioration usually imply that mental disorder produces a lowering in the level of cognitive ability. The vocabularly test is used to estimate past level, and non-vocabulary tests are used to estimate present cognitive level. The discrepancy between these two measures is usually taken as an index of the patient's deterioration. This kind of index was first developed by Babcock. It should be remembered, however, that Babcock also suggested that the cognitive deterioration of psychiatric patients might consist of a discrepancy between present level and present speed of function and she expected her index to measure this discrepancy as well. It has been demonstrated elsewhere (*5, 10*) that Babcock did not provide unequivocal evidence for her theories. The evidence reported in this paper is in effect, the beginning of the provision of such evidence.

Third, it would seem that the outcome of the investigation reported in this paper, confirms the soundness of the methodological conceptions described at the outset. The investigation of a single aspect of psychological function on a single case does not necessarily bog down the investigator amongst a mass of unrelatable observations, so long as the investigation is linked from the very first with the aim of explanation, and so long as the attempt is made to check every explanation by controlled observation. With this precaution, the investigation of the single case can lead to discoveries of general significance.

This conclusion does not imply that the psychologist must always start from scratch. It is obviously better to take validated descriptive generalizations about psychiatric patients as starting points of investigations, if they are available. Even then, it would probably be necessary to return frequently to the single case investigation, at various stages of the development of a research project. The validity of this last proposition, however, still remains to be tested.

Finally, we have to consider how far we have gone in the explanation of the initial observation: the patient's inability to comprehend simple material when read aloud. It would seem that in the first place this difficulty is shared by many normal people of above average ability. It does not, however, exist to the same degree among them as it did in our patient.

The greater degree of difficulty shown by our patient may be due to two reasons. First, the patient's relative slowness of reading might have made it more difficult for him to comprehend what he read. A certain minimum rate of reading might be necessary to facilitate comprehension. In the second place, the patient's rate of comprehension might have been too slow for even his rate of reading aloud. The need to test these two hypotheses is emphasized by the fact that the patient showed no difficulty of comprehension in the silent reading test, providing he was given enough time. This might mean, in accordance with the first theory, that he had in this situation the opportunity of going over the material more than once, or, in accordance with the second theory, the opportunity of reading at his own rate of comprehension. The extent to which the two explanations were correct could only be determined by experiment, and this we did not have the opportunity of doing.

The more general complaint of the patient, his inability to complete the reading of a book, has not of course been finally explained. It might well be that his slowness of performance made it difficult for him to comprehend the main burden of what he was reading and, therefore, he became lost and had to give up the task. A detailed investigation of his reading activity would have been necessary to clear up this matter. It suffices for the purpose of this paper, merely to note that despite the final incompleteness of the investigation, we had arrived at generalities of some importance, both to the patient himself and to clinical psychology in general.

SUMMARY

This paper gives an account of the application of the single case method in the opening up of a field of research in clinical psychology. The investigation results in drawing attention to, and providing confirmation of, one of Babcock's conceptions of deterioration, which has recently suffered some neglect. This is to the effect that cooperative psychotic patients may be very slow in the carrying out of cognitive operations without suffering much loss in the level of difficulty they attain when given sufficient time.

REFERENCES

1. Burt, C. *Mental and scholastic tests.* London: Staples Press, 1947.
2. Eysenck, H. J. *Differential cognitive tests.* In: U.S. Navy Contract No. N625585-56, 1953.
3. Furneaux, W. D. Some speed, error and difficulty relationships within a problem solving situation. *Nature,* 1952, 170, 37.
4. Furneaux, W. D. *A note on the "Nufferno" tests of inductive reasoning abilities, including summaries of such norms as have so far been established. Part 2. Speed. The S. E. Tests.* 1953 (Unpublished paper).
5. Nelson, E. H. *An experimental investigation of intellectual speed and power in mental disorders.* Ph.D. Thesis, Univ. London, 1953.
6. Ogilvie, B. C. *A study of intellectual slowness in schizophrenia.* Ph.D. Thesis, Univ. London, 1953.
7. Schonell, F. J. and Schonell, F. E. *Diagnostic and attainment testing.* London: Oliver & Boyd, 1950.
8. Shapiro, M. B. Experimental studies of a perceptual anomaly. I. Initial experiments. *J. Ment. Sci.,* 1951, *97,* 90–110.
9. Shapiro, M. B. Experimental studies of a perceptual anomaly. II. Confirmatory and explanatory experiments. *J. Ment. Sci.,* 1952, *98,* 605–617.
10. Shapiro, M. B. Use of psychological tests for the differential diagnosis of early dementia. *Proc. Roy. Soc. Med.,* 1952, *45,* 375–376.
11. Shapiro, M. B. Experimental studies of a perceptual anomaly. III. The testing of an explanatory theory. *J. Ment. Sci.,* 1953, *99,* 394–409.

8

Speed of Function and Educational Retardation: The Psychological and Psychiatric Investigation of an Individual Case*

A. T. RAVENETTE and L. A. HERSOV

1. INTRODUCTION

Investigation of children at child guidance clinics commonly falls into three parts: social, psychiatric and psychological. Whilst the inter-relatedness of the social and psychiatric findings is usually quite clear, the findings of the psychologist often tend to be additional, rather than related, to the other findings—unless his results arise from the use of projective techniques. This division is further reinforced by the fact that the psychologist's contribution is usually restricted to the first diagnostic interview and thereafter the patient's handling is carried on by the other members of the clinic team. It occasionally happens, however, that the preliminary investigation raises issues which call for more intensive exploration by the psychologist, and when this happens there is need for close co-operation between psychologist and psychiatrist in order to formulate more precisely an individual child's disability. This paper provides an example of such collaboration in an intensive psychological investigation, the final conclusions of which could only be reached by evaluating psychological findings in the light of psychiatric findings collated from previous and current records.

* Reprinted from the *Journal of Child Psychology and Psychiatry*, 1963, Vol. 4, pp. 17–28, by permission of the authors and the publisher.

Communicating such a case, however, raises a difficult problem. Psychiatric presentation is considerably different in style and content from that of a psychologist. Whereas the former is of necessity historic and descriptive, the latter attempts an exposition of experimental work involving methodological argument and statistical tables. To give equal emphasis to each in one paper would lead to excessive length and diffuseness. Alternatively, if the paper were reduced to manageable proportions neither argument would be given sufficient space for its adequate development. In the present circumstances it was considered appropriate to present the psychiatric aspects of the case in as concise and abbreviated a manner as possible, thereby allowing a full presentation of the psychological investigations. The decision was made since, from a purely psychological point of view, this case suggests a number of important methodological and theoretical issues.

The psychological investigation of the single case is often a necessity, e.g. Shapiro and Nelson (1955), Bartlett and Shapiro (1956), Shapiro and Ravenette (1959) and Shapiro (1961). Standardized tests provide useful, if limited, information, but they are seldom suitable to test specific hypotheses concerning an individual patient. It becomes necessary, therefore, to devise objective means of investigation specifically related to the case in hand. Whilst this may frequently be time-consuming, it has the advantage of suggesting ideas of greater generality as well as providing answers to the immediate problems. The particular issues arising from this case will be discussed at the end of the paper.

2. THE PROBLEM

Robert, the elder of two brothers, now aged 10 years, had been referred to child guidance clinics as an infant. In a follow-up survey his mother asked for help as he had made unsatisfactory progress in school, especially in arithmetic. The problem for the psychologist was to elucidate the facts of the case, to establish causes, if possible, and to suggest remedies. The problem for the psychiatrist was to view the present situation in the light of the boy's previous history, and to assess the relevance of personality factors acting on the child's educational and cognitive performances. In seeking a solution which did justice to all the information the psychologist and psychiatrist were inevitably brought into very close co-operation.

Clinical History

Robert was referred to child guidance clinics at the age of three years by his family doctor. The symptoms were restlessness, stubbornness, disobedience, lack of regard for his safety and refusal to play with other children. He also walked with an unsteady gait, frequently fell down and was subject to "blank spells" lasting for about a minute, but without incontinence or lack of consciousness. Poor motor development had been noticeable from the age of 1 year. In a personal communication, the family doctor reported that the pregnancy was normal apart from persistent nausea and vomiting, which did not require hospitalization. The birth in a nursing home was normal.

Testing on the Merrill Palmer Intelligence Test gave Robert an I.Q. of 89. This was considered an underestimate because of his distractibility, refusal of items and lack of acknowledgment of verbal instructions in the test situation. A skull X-ray showed no abnormality. In the psychiatric interviews he became increasingly restless and distractible and eventually it was impossible to command his attention.

Within the family situation the mother was tense, over-anxious and protective, whilst the father, the manager of a departmental store, was firm to the extent of being punitive. The differences between the parents over the boy's management had led to a considerable strain in the marriage relationship.

At 3 years 6 months an E.E.G. showed a doubtful excess of fast activity but no other abnormality. Brain damage was considered but discounted in the absence of supporting evidence. During the next 18 months the boy attended the clinic for "play therapy" and the problems of management were discussed with both parents. The treatment resulted in more consistent handling by the parents and when it finished at the age of 4 years 6 months Robert was considered to be much improved with respect to his distractibility, hyperkinesis and co-ordination of movement and speech. Re-testing with the Stanford Binet Intelligence Scale at this age gave Robert an I.Q. of 92.

Description of the Situation at the Time of Follow-up

The mother's main concern was Robert's failure to make satisfactory progress at school. He was extremely slow in his written work, especially in arithmetic, and in such activities he daydreamed, had "blank spells" and was usually "miles away." Other complaints were of occasional diarrhoea before going to school, temper tantrums, inability to play with other children of his own age or to withstand teasing and rough games. He was also solitary and depressed at times. On the positive side distractibility and restlessness were no longer considered by the mother to be serious and he also showed fair aptitude for mechanical and constructional toys.

The mother's concern over the boy's failure in school had led to arguments with the head teachers at the three schools which he had attended. At the same time she exerted considerable pressure on Robert at home towards achievement and to this end had also engaged a tutor for evening coaching.

In the psychiatric interview Robert was cheerful and talkative and very interested in the toys, objects and apparatus in the office. He repeatedly asked intelligent questions about how things worked and their use. When, however, the topic of school progress was introduced he became miserable and downcast. He was reluctant to answer questions and frequently tried to bring the conversation back to earlier topics.

A report from his present head teacher described his attainment as follows:

Arithmetic. Very weak, seems unable to grasp the simplest principles.

Written English. Achieves very little, seems to find difficulty in concentrating for more than a few minutes.

General. . . . very slow in all things . . . lacks muscular control, especially in handwriting.

It was also reported that in the 9 plus selection tests, Robert's Moray House (No. 55) I.Q. was 92.

3. PRELIMINARY PSYCHOLOGICAL TESTING

W.I.S.C. FULL SCALE I.Q. 117

Verbal Scale I.Q.	124	*Performance Scale I.Q.*	106
Comprehension	13	Picture Completion	11
Arithmetic	14	Picture Arrangement	8
Similarities	14	Block Design	15
Vocabulary	15	Object Assembly	15
Digit Span	13	Coding	5

Reading Age (Schonell Graded Word Reading Test) 13. 1 years.
Arithmetic Age Schonell Essential Arithmetic Test, 9 years 10 months
Schonell Diagnostic Arithmetic Test No. 5, 9 years 6 months
Schonell Diagnostic Arithmetic Test No. 12, 10 years 2 months.

In view of the reports of poor muscular co-ordination the Oseretsky Scale of Motor Proficiency (Doll, 1946) was administered. It was recognized that the standardization data for this test were not necessarily satisfactory but it was considered that it should provide some useful information about this aspect of the boy's development.

Level of motor development
General Static 8½ years.
Dynamic Manual 8½ years.
General Dynamic 9 years.
Simultaneous Movement 8½ years.
Speed 5 years.
Asynkinesia 8 years.

Discussion of Results

Intelligence. No data is available to compare directly the Stanford Binet I.Q. at the age of 4½ years (92) and the present W.I.S.C. I.Q. (117). Thorndyke (1933), however, suggests a correlation of 0.698 between test and retest over 5 months on the Stanford Binet. A correlation of this order gives a Standard Error of Prediction of 10.6 I.Q. points and consequently a retest I.Q. of 117 would have a chance probability of less than 1 per cent. Moreover the reliability figures for the W.I.S.C. Full Scale I.Q.

($SE_E = 3.36$) indicate that Robert's true I.Q. would fall between 110 and 124 95 per cent of the times on retest. It seems reasonable to suppose therefore that the W.I.S.C. assessment indicates a reliable increase of measured intelligence. The explanation of this increase is likely to be twofold. In the first place the evidence of Robert's poor testability as an infant suggests that the test results at the time may well be underestimates. Secondly, as Gunzburg (1958) says, the Stanford Binet test has a marked performance loading at the lower age range. In view of the boy's history of poor motor ability, this would affect his intelligence assessment at the age of 5 years.

The W.I.S.C. result shows a discrepancy of 18 points between the verbal and performance scales. Using the methods suggested by Payne and Jones (1957), it can be determined that such a discrepancy occurred in 7½ per cent of the standardization population and would occur due to errors of measurement less than 5 per cent of the time on successive retesting. The discrepancy, however, really rests on the poor Picture Arrangement and Coding subtest scores. Using a technique adapted by Maxwell (personal communication) from Scheffé (1953) the difference between the mean of these two tests and the mean of other performance sub-tests is statistically significant at the 1 per cent level.

The I.Q. of 92 on the Moray House Test is comparable to the test results in infancy and with the measured arithmetic attainment. It is however at variance with the W.I.S.C. assessment which is considered to be reliable. It should be noted that this test is a paper and pencil test of verbal reasoning which involves answering a large number of questions in a fairly short time and is therefore considerably weighted in favour of speed.

Motor development. According to the normative data provided with the Oseretsky Scale these results indicate a mild degree of general retardation but serious retardation in motor speed. Whilst it is accepted that the overall norms may be unsatisfactory it would seem reasonable to allow internal consistency to obtain between the six sub-scales. Consequently this evidence of differential motor development is considered to be acceptable. Poor motor speed would be reflected in the school situation in speed of writing and in handwriting skills generally.

Educational attainment. Robert's reading attainment is consistent with his general level of verbal ability. The arithmetic scores are, however, somewhat anomalous when compared with the other evidence. No data is available to indicate the range of arithmetic attainment normally associated with a given intelligence level, but using Schonell's (1942) criterion of 1½–2 years retardation from general ability level, these attainment scores do indicate sufficient retardation to be considered serious. There appears however to be a large discrepancy between Robert's attainment in school ("seems unable to grasp the simplest principles") and his attainment in the clinic situation ("Arithmetic Age" 9.10 years). Moreover there appears to be a similar discrepancy between these tests and the mental arithmetic level indicated on the W.I.S.C. (Test Age 12.6 years).

It was noticed during the arithmetic tests that he made no computational errors but he did take a very long time in writing down his answers. When questioned about this he said that he was making sure that his answer was correct. He was also easily distracted by objects in the environment.

Reformulation of the Problem

Robert, at the time of investigation, is therefore a boy of bright average and in many respects superior intelligence. Despite this, his measured arithmetic attainment on written standardized tests is consistent with that of a boy of only average intelligence. In this sense he can be considered retarded in arithmetic. Nonetheless, on the one hand his Test Age on the Arithmetic sub-test of the W.I.S.C. is 12½-years, indicating above-average ability in mental arithmetic when no writing is involved, and on the other hand he is reported to be unable to grasp the simplest principles in school. It would seem then that the retardation is not in arithmetic *per se,* but in showing that he can satisfactorily complete an arithmetic exercise in school or an attainment test.

In the light of Robert's intelligence level the following weaknesses seem to be relevant:

1. Poor Coding, and possibly poor Picture Arrangement ability.
2. Poor performance on the Moray House Test.

3. Not higher than average attainment on standardized tests of arithmetic, the main features being his high accuracy and low speed.
4. Poor motor speed as measured by the Oseretsky Scale.

The common factor to each of the first three points is speed of functioning. This speed can be either motor (as involved in writing answers) or cognitive, i.e. working out the correct solution in his head. It is therefore postulated that Robert's disability results from either: (1) Poor motor speed (for which the Oseretsky results and the psychiatric history give some support) or, (2) poor cognitive speed or, (3) a combination of poor motor and poor cognitive speed.

As no standardized tests are available which could be used to test these hypotheses it becomes necessary to set up an experimental investigation directly related to this particular problem.

A further line of enquiry is suggested by the W.I.S.C./Moray House discrepancy. A re-test on the same Moray House test would give further information as to the importance of the speed factor in a test situation extended over 30 min. It was proposed therefore to re-test Robert as soon as possible, but actually this could not be done until after the other investigations had been completed.

4. EXPERIMENTAL INVESTIGATION OF THE RELATIVE CONTRIBUTION OF MOTOR AND COGNITIVE SPEED IN TESTS OF SIMPLE ARITHMETIC BONDS

The work of Furneaux (1952) suggests that when speed is the variable to be measured it is important not to mix together times for correct and incorrect solutions to problems. It follows from this that the arithmetic given should be well within Robert's range of ability. The choice of material was, therefore, addition and subtraction bonds similar to those given in the Schonell Diagnostic Arithmetic Test No. 5, e.g. $8 + 4$, $16 - 8$. All these bonds were demonstrably within Robert's level of ability.

Such tests can be given visually, as in the Schonell tests, or verbally. In order to reduce the number of variables and to give maximum accuracy of timing, the verbal method was used. This avoids having to make an allowance for reading time, and enables timing to commence from the moment the instruction is given. The test then involves two specific abilities: (a) speed of solving a sum, and (b) speed of writing the answer.

In order to obtain separate measures of each it is necessary to record the time taken to write numbers only and this time can be subtracted from the writing plus solving time to give a measure of solving time only. Alternatively, if the subject gives his answer verbally, instead of writing it down, the time recorded for his answer is substantially a measure of solving time. In the outcome the latter method was used for analysis as it appeared to be the more reliable.

Bearing these considerations in mind the investigation was planned in the following manner. The test involved:

1. Solving and writing down the answers to addition and subtraction bonds given verbally.
2. Writing down numbers as dictated. These numbers were the same as the answers in (1) above.
3. Solving the same sums but giving the answers verbally.

There were eight addition and eight subtraction bonds. The former gave the answers from 2 to 9 and the latter gave the answers from 10 to 16. (Through error two sums were given to which the answer was 10.) The bonds were obtained by using a table of random numbers. Distribution of bonds and digits throughout the test was randomized by means of a Latin square. To avoid confusion to Robert during the experiment, the written test was given first and the test requiring a verbal answer followed. All responses were timed and timing commenced after the sum or number had been stated.

As this test material was designed to be comparable to the Schonell Diagnostic Arithmetic tests it should be possible to make certain predictions concerning the relative contributions of writing and solving speeds involved in such tests. Normative data is available whereby an attainment age is given according to the number of sums correctly answered in a given time. If this procedure is valid it must rest on the assumption that most of the time is used in working out the solution and only a small amount of time is used in recording the answer. In other words, variations in measured attainment should reflect variations in cognitive speed. The prediction, therefore, in the case of Robert is that, if he is normal with respect to speed, his "writing plus solving" time ($w + s$) would be greater than "solving" time (s) which would in turn be greater than "writing" time (w), and that the difference between w and s would be statistically significant. Any other relationship between w and s would indicate that in this type of task the greater determinant of success in a timed written test would be speed of writing, i.e. motor speed.

Results and discussion. As response times were positively skewed it was necessary to carry out a logarithmic transformation in order to normalize the data. Using analysis of variance, it was found that the mean log ($w + s$) was 0.523, the mean log w was 0.282 and the mean log s was 0.328; s was significantly less than ($w + s$) ($t = 2.7$ with 15 *d.f.* $p < 0.01$) but the difference between s and w failed to reach an acceptable level of significance ($t = 1.0$).

It follows from our argument, therefore, that the time Robert spends in writing his answers is too great, i.e. his motor speed is a handicap. This supports the hypothesis that his difficulties arise from poor motor speed.

It is not sufficient, however, to leave the investigation at this stage since it is not known how children who are considered to be normal would perform in this situation. The testing of a control sample is necessary in order to validate the assumption concerning the relative importance of motor and cognitive speed and to relate Robert's performance to that of normals.

Investigation with Control Subjects

Six boys were selected from Robert's school, three in the "A" stream and three in the "B" stream. The basis for selection was that they should be of comparable age and general intelligence. It was known that most "A" and "B" stream children would be selected for either grammar or technical school education (i.e. were of bright average or higher ability), and the boys in the "C" stream on balance would be of lower intelligence than

Robert. The identical tests were given to each child and for the purpose of statistical analysis Robert's results were included with theirs (cf. Maxwell, 1958).

Results and discussion. Because of the rapidity of the children's responses it was necessary to add a constant before carrying out the logarithmic transformation. A method elaborated by Duncan (1955)[1] was used to compare the means after analysis of variance.

1. Solving times (s). Analysis of variance showed that the differences between children were highly significant ($F = 3.9$ with 6 *d.f.* $p < 0.01$). The mean log time scores are given in Table 1.

Differences between items were also highly significant ($F = 3.1$ with 15 *d.f.* $p < 0.001$) and these differences were related to the difficulty level of number bonds where either the answer, or part of the question, involved numbers greater than 10.

2. Writing times (w). Analysis of variance showed that the differences between children were highly significant ($F = 28.4$ with 6 *d.f.* $p < 0.001$) but the differences between items were not significant ($F = 0.75$). The mean log time scores are given in Table 2.

It is clear that the third of our hypotheses is the relevant one, i.e. Robert's disability is one of both motor and cognitive slowness. (It is worth noting that the sixth boy in Table 2 is significantly slower than the other controls but there was no suggestion that he was presenting problems in school achievement.)

School Visit

The visit to test the control sample at Robert's school provided an opportunity to obtain more information about the school and about Robert himself. It was reported that Robert was in the "C" stream and that there was no evidence in his school work to justify promotion. It was perhaps unfortunate that Robert's

[1] This technique allows for the fact that when n mean scores are available there are ${}_nC_2$ ways of choosing any two scores. This must be taken into account when tests of significance are carried out. Rp is a function of the *range* between *means* (when these are ordered by magnitude), the degrees of freedom of the residual from the analysis of variance and the standard error of the mean. Numerical values for computing Rp are given in Duncan's paper.

TABLE 1

Mean Log Solving Times of Subjects

Subject	1	2	3	4	5	6	7
Mean Log Time	0·286	0·302	0·312	0·322	0·386	0·390	0·646
Difference		0·016	0·010	0·010	0·064	0·004	0·256

At 1 per cent level of significance $Rp=0{\cdot}236$, hence difference between means of Nos. 6 and 7 (Robert) is significant at the 0·01 level.

TABLE 2

Mean Log Solving Times of Subjects

Subject	1	2	3	4	5	6	7
Mean Log Writing Time	0·306	0·312	0·319	0·333	0·342	0·446	0·592
Difference		0·006	0·007	0·014	0·009	0·124	0·146

At 1 per cent level of significance $Rp=0{\cdot}055$, hence differences between means of Nos. 5 and 6 and Nos. 6 and 7 (Robert) are significant at the 0·01 level.

teacher was young and inexperienced. The school itself is in a very good class residential area and the standards are very high as it is only the "C" stream children who fail to be selected for grammar or technical school education.

Moray House Test Results

Some time after Robert had started attending the clinic for investigation he had taken a further Moray House Verbal Reasoning Test (No. 56) and on this occasion he obtained an I.Q. of 106. When he was again retested on the Moray House Test he gained an I.Q. of 115, within the prescribed time (39 min.). He was allowed to finish the test and in an extra 10 min. made four more correct responses giving an equivalent I.Q. of 117. His total number of errors was 50 out of 107.

The three test results, with a three-month gap between each test, are 92, 106 and 115, giving a gain of 23 points in 6 months. No correlational data was available to assess the statistical significance of this gain directly, but Peel (1951) in his work on Moray House re-testing argues that a gain of about 5 points could be expected over four weeks. A second re-test, however, tends to show little further improvement. The first gain therefore of 14 points is unlikely to be within normal retest limits and the further gain of 9 points even less so. It is possible that situational factors played a big part in the final re-test, e.g. no competitive feelings, minimal distraction, and personal contact with the tester. This suggestion is consistent with the more general finding of Yates (1953) that a considerable proportion of children who make disproportionate gains on group tests do so because their initial score is depressed by "lack of incentive, illness, anxiety, emotional disturbance or conflict."

5. SUMMARY OF PSYCHOLOGICAL AND PSYCHIATRIC FINDINGS: POSSIBLE EXPLANATIONS

The threads of these investigations now need to be drawn together. Over and above the initial data the following findings emerge:

1. Motor retardation, especially in motor speed.
2. Cognitive slowness in arithmetic and probably in all school subjects.
3. Disproportionate increases in Moray House I.Q. over a period of six months.
4. With the Moray House Test given under ideal conditions, an I.Q. is obtained which approximates to the verbal I.Q. obtained on the W.I.S.C.

These findings need to be related to the clinical picture built up over the years.

The salient points of Robert's development are:

1. Poor motor development from the age of 1 year.
2. Robert's mother was disappointed with the boy as he grew up because he did not measure up to her expectations. Consequently she simultaneously made excessive demands on him and became oversolicitous for him.
3. The father adopted an attitude opposed to that of the mother which resulted in inconsistent handling.
4. At the age of 2½–5 Robert showed a clinical picture of hyperactivity, distractibility and poor concentration which has been considered by some to be the consequence of brain damage (Laufer, Denhoff and Solomons, 1957). An E.E.G. at the time was suggestive, but not typical, of brain damage, but there were no neurological signs nor was there anything in the pregnancy and birth history to support such an hypothesis.
5. From the age of 5 years the hyperkinetic syndrome gradually improved with better handling by the mother, but she remained very anxious and became even more so as Robert failed to make progress at school.
6. In spite of the overall improvement in hyperkinesis, during the current test sessions Robert was noticeably distractible and extremely talkative. Any unusual object, e.g. a stop-watch, was the occasion for exhaustive questioning. He wanted to know all the details and as much of the mechanism and purpose as possible.

Two possible explanations can be suggested to fit these findings. The first is in terms of brain damage and the second is in terms of reaction to stress. A third possibility is that a combination of both is the correct explanation.

Brain Damage

Motor retardation may well be a direct result of brain damage. Cognitive slowness and his very poor school record could be explained by Robert's distractibility and his obsessional checking. The final Moray House I.Q. obtained in physical conditions, comparable to those prescribed by Strauss and Lehtinen (1947) for the education of brain-damaged children, would not unexpectedly approximate to the I.Q. obtained on the W.I.S.C.

The evidence to support this hypothesis is the clinical picture shown by Robert as an infant and his present distractibility and mild hyperkinesis.

A further E.E.G. investigation was requested to test this hypothesis but the E.E.G. was completely normal. The hypothesis was therefore considered not proven.

Reaction to Stress and Parental Handling

The two significant factors in this explanation are (a) the motor retardation (which may be maturational) and (b) the attitude of the mother (indicated above). The clinical picture at 5 years could then be explained as the child's reactions to the parents' attitudes and the mother's demands. As this behaviour improved with improved parental handling the motor retardation remained, but this time its effect was now most evident in the school situation. Failure, occasioned by his motor handicap, led to a heightening of maternal concern and therefore more stress. This gave rise to anxiety, meticulous checking, and, with continued failure, an escape from work by means of day-dreaming. All of this is consistent with the observed cognitive slowness and the school report of day-dreaming. It is not surprising that when the Moray House Test was given under the most favourable conditions, i.e. least stressful, he obtained so high a score.

This formulation, it was felt, accounted most adequately for all the data and, moreover, would obtain equally well even if Robert was minimally brain-damaged. Recommendations were made, therefore, to those responsible for Robert's further education in the light of this formulation.

6. THEORETICAL DISCUSSION

This investigation has thrown up a number of issues which are both theoretically and practically interesting. In the first place, the only proof that an individual has learned something occurs in the performance or recounting of what has been learned. When, as in the case presented here, an individual gives no evidence in school of learning, it is not necessarily unreasonable to assume that he cannot or has been unable to learn. Nonetheless, Robert, who in the school situation could be labelled "retarded," in the individual test situation shows arithmetical ability commensurate with his intellectual ability. Whilst it is not argued that such a disparity in performance is common in the general population, it would seem worthwhile to ascertain how many so-called "retarded" children are, indeed, "pseudo-retarded."

Secondly, much of this paper has been concerned with speed of function in carrying out simple arithmetical operations. This topic has not, to the authors' knowledge, been examined in this way before, and it would seem, in the light of the findings reported here that motor and cognitive speed are important variables affecting an individual's performance. Research into these variables might be extremely useful in assessing educational weaknesses.

Thirdly, the research of Nelson (1953) and Nelson and Shapiro (1955) in the field of adult psychiatric groups provides a parallel set of findings to those reported in this paper. They found that cognitively, the most important distinguishing characteristic between normal adults and adults in various psychiatric groups was slowness of mental functioning. Over and above this, however, within these psychiatric groups there could be distinguished two relatively independent factors—motor and mental speed. It is not argued that what is true for adults is necessarily true for children, but nonetheless the parallel is suggestive.

Fourthly, it has often been noticed that the coding subtest score tends to be low for clinic tested children, and Maxwell (1961) provides evidence confirming this observation. In that this test is quite closely related to some aspects of school work it does not seem to be unreasonable to argue that a low score reflects anxiety in the school situation, or poor motor speed, since the test is a pencil and paper one, and that a very low score reflects the additive effect of both factors. This hypothesis may well be too simple but it would be well worth investigating.

Finally, there is the general question of what, over and above manifest content, tests really measure. Our control subjects' results suggest that under certain circumstances a test of arithmetic is measuring motor speed (cf. Tables 1 and 2) just as much as cognitive speed and accuracy. It is necessary to know just what the variables are that determine a test score, and the relationship between them, at different age levels, and at different levels of ability. It might then be possible to construct unidimensional scales the validity of which is far more accurately known.

Conclusions

A case of this type is comparatively rare in that information from other clinics was available to cover most of the boy's life. Moreover it is not always possible to carry out so full a psychological investigation as was possible in this case. The outcome of the investigation suggests that Robert's present failure in school arises from causes operating in early life, namely, his motor slowness and the mother's high expectations of him. The change from behaviour disorder in infancy to inadequate achievement in school is in itself interesting. Whilst the former improved, the latter did not become manifest for some considerable time. This delay is not surprising as Robert changed schools so many times, and comparative failure in any one school could be attributed to a failure to settle down. His move to his present school, however, with its very high standards, probably accentuated Robert's difficulties and made his disability more obvious. Had he moved to a school with lesser educational demands he would probably have attracted much less attention and indeed might well have shown himself capable of performing educationally at a level much more comparable to his intellectual ability.

7. SUMMARY

This paper reports the psychological and psychiatric investigation of a 10-year-old boy referred to the Clinic for backwardness at school, especially in arithmetic. In the outcome it was found that Robert was severely handicapped both in motor speed and speed of cognitive functioning. It was argued that the boy's observed difficulties in school arose from his motor handicap and his reactions to parental pressure for achievement. Certain theoretical issues are also discussed arising from this investigation.

REFERENCES

BARTLETT, D. and SHAPIRO, M. B. (1956) Investigation and treatment of a reading disability in a dull child with a severe psychiatric disturbance. *Brit. J. educ. Psychol. 24,* 180–190.

DOLL, E. A. (1946) *Manual for the Oseretsky Motor Proficiency Tests.* C. H. Stoelting, Chicago.

DUNCAN, D. B. (1955) Multiple Range and Multiple *F* tests. *Biometrics. 11,* 1–42.

FURNEAUX, W. D. (1952) Some speed, error and difficulty relationships within a problem solving situation. *Nature, Lond. 170,* 37–39.

GUNZBURG, H. C. (1958) Psychological Assessment in mental deficiency. In *Mental Deficiency: the changing outlook.* (Edited by CLARKE, ANNE M. and CLARKE, A. D. B.) Methuen, London.

LAUFER, M. W., DENHOFF, E. E. and SOLOMONS, G. (1957) Hyperkinetic impulse disorder in children's behaviour problems. *Psychosom. Med. 19,* 38–54.

MAXWELL, A. E. (1958) *Experimental Design in Psychology and the Medical Science.* Methuen, London.

MAXWELL, A. E. (1961) Discrepancies between the pattern of abilities for normal and neurotic children. *J. ment. Sci. 107,* 300–307.

Moray House Tests (1957) University of London Press. (These are closed tests not available to the public.)

NELSON, E. H. (1953) An experimental investigation of intellectual speed and power in mental disorders. Unpublished Ph.D. thesis University of London Library.

NELSON, E. H. and SHAPIRO, M. B. (1955) An investigation of the nature of cognitive impairment in co-operative psychiatric patients. *Brit. J. med. Psychol. 28,* 239–256.

PAYNE, R. W. and JONES, H. G. (1957) Statistics for the investigation of the individual case. *J. clin. Psychol. 23,* 115–121.

PEEL, E. A. (1951) A note on practice effects in intelligence tests. *Brit. J. educ. Psychol. 21,* 122–126.

SCHEFFE, A. (1953) A method for judging all contrasts in the analysis of variance. *Biometrika. 40,* 87–104.

SCHONELL, F. J. (1942) *Backwardness in the Basic Subjects.* Oliver and Boyd, Edinburgh.

SHAPIRO, M. B. (1961) The Single Case in fundamental clinical psychological research. *Brit. J. med. Psychol. 34,* 255–262.

SHAPIRO, M. B. and NELSON, E. H. (1955) An investigation of an abnormality of cognitive functioning in a co-operative young psychotic: an example of the application of experimental method to the single case. *J. clin. Psychol. 11,* 344–351.

SHAPIRO, M. B. and RAVENETTE, A. T. (1959) A preliminary experiment on paranoid delusions. *J. ment. Sci. 105,* 295–312.

STRAUSS, A. A. and LEHTINEN, L. E. (1947) *Psychopathology and education of the brain injured child.* Grune and Stratton, New York.

THORNDIKE, R. L. (1933) The effect of the interval between test and re-test on the constancy of the I.Q. *J. educ. Psychol. 24,* 543–549.

YATES, A. (1953) Symposium on the effects of coaching and practice in intelligence tests. An analysis of some recent investigations. *Brit. J. educ. Psychol. 23,* 147–154.

9

Demonstration of a Psychosomatic Relationship*

Maryse Metcalfe

An illness cannot be assumed to be psychosomatic until it has been demonstrated objectively that physical events which are part of that illness, tend to occur after or in conjunction with psychological events of a particular nature. This might in theory be demonstrated by three different methods: firstly by studying the emotional events associated with the beginning of the illness or with its recurrence; secondly by measuring those underlying physiological changes relevant to that illness which accompany or follow specific emotional changes; and thirdly by describing as many as possible of the emotional and relevant physical changes over a period of time for a single individual and attempting to find out how they relate to each other.

The latter method appears particularly suitable to the study of asthma. Here the attack is a dramatic enough event to be directly observed and recorded and the physical end of the connexion can thus be easily assessed. But the emotional event which precedes it is obviously more difficult to detect; it is never simple to obtain an objective reporting of emotional states whether through introspection or from an outside observer. Alexander & French (1941) rightly point out in their monograph that those emotional events which they believe to be associated with the occurrence of the asthmatic attacks may well have been directly conditioned by the analytical situation itself; this would partly explain the importance given to conflicts about dependence. In the absence of direct assessment of emotion one can consider, instead of the emotion proper, certain well-defined and observ-

* Reprinted from the *British Journal of Medical Psychology,* 1956, Vol. 29, pp. 63–66, by permission of the author and the publisher.

able environmental situations which are presumably related to the specific emotion. The following study is an attempt to demonstrate a relationship between attacks and an objective and well-defined situation which was assumed to possess an important emotional loading for the patient.

PERSONAL HISTORY

An unmarried girl aged 21 had been sent to the Maudsley Hospital by her industrial physician because her job was in jeopardy owing to frequent absences with attacks of asthma.

She had developed asthma at the age of 5 following frequent colds. Her schooling was interrupted by frequent attacks which often lasted for three weeks. From 7 to 15 she was evacuated from London and lived with a foster-mother away from her family. Her attacks continued, but in the last year of that period she had improved greatly and was mostly free of them. She then returned to her own home in London and her attacks immediately started again, reaching a peak of intensity when she was 19. For the two years prior to her admission to hospital she had been improving but had suffered three severe attacks, each lasting two or three weeks and also a mild attack every morning during the whole of the two years. In addition to the asthma she complained of frontal and temporal throbbing headaches which occasionally culminated in vomiting. At the time of her admission she was living at home with her mother. The father, a drunkard who gambled, swore and quarrelled with everyone, had left home two years previously. In the home there also lived her mother's lover, and her father's adoptive father.

The patient was a well-developed girl with mild acne on her face and neck. There was no physical abnormality in any system. She was active, cheerful, but was subject to occasional bouts of irritability and depression. Her intelligence was below average (Progressive Matrices I.Q. 89, Wechsler-Bellevue I.Q. 82). She was quite successful in her job as a hairdresser, although she was in conflict there with her immediate superior—a woman whom she disliked intensely and towards whom she was rude and aggressive. Superficially sociable, she had no intimate friends and her hobby of ballroom dancing was her main interest. She professed to not set purpose in life.

For her asthma she had been referred to an allergist at the age of 16; skin tests had shown a positive reaction to house dust, beef and pork, but she had received no specific treatment. She herself had not asked to see a psychiatrist and had been surprised when her physician had recommended her to do so.

CLINICAL FORMULATION

When the clinical investigations were completed the following formulation was made by the psychiatrist. "The attacks of asthma could result in this patient from several stimuli, physical ones (allergens, infections) or emotional disturbances. The key figure in her life was her mother to whom she had ambivalent feelings. When asthmatic attacks resulted from emotional disturbances this disturbance was connected with the mother. The attacks were most probably an expression of her inhibited aggression. Free ventilation of the patient's hostile feelings both generally and more specifically toward her mother would lead to their modification and hence to a diminution in the frequency or severity (or both) of her attacks."

Attempt to Start an Attack Experimentally

Initially an effort was made to precipitate an attack by presenting the patient with emotional stimuli connected with her mother. These consisted of T.A.T., Rorschach cards, and words related to mother. This experimental approach was based on the claim made by clinicians that an attack can be started in an asthmatic by subjecting him to a specific emotional stress. But the approach failed here and the patient never developed an attack under those conditions.

Interviews

It was then decided to turn to a passive method of recording as many observations as possible of the patient's daily life. This was linked with interviews aimed at ventilating her feelings.

The patient was interviewed 66 times over a period of 85 days. Those interviews were recorded in full, the interviewing psychologist maintaining a friendly but passive attitude throughout. For the longest part of the interview the patient was asked to speak freely on a series of selected topics. Each was selected by the psychologist prior to the interview; the topics chosen were Mother, Father, Foster-mother, Grandfather, Step-father, Sex and Work. But at the beginning of each interview, the patient, who was keeping a detailed day-to-day diary, reported on all her symptoms, moods and reactions. A record was made of all these variables.

Each daily recording included:

(*a*) All symptoms related to respiration. These were of two sorts, the first a fleeting wheezing or tightness of the chest, which the patient dismissed as "not real asthma." Then there were the "real" asthmatic attacks. These consisted of tightness, wheezing and severe respiratory distress. The present study is only concerned with these to the exclusion of all other physical symptoms. These attacks occurred on 15 days of the 85 she spent in hospital.

(*b*) Other physical symptoms not related to respiration. The patient complained of sixteen mild symptoms (headaches, etc.) throughout her stay.

(*c*) All her activities, such as games, dancing, occupational therapy, shopping expeditions, meetings with her mother and visits to her home or to friends' homes. She also reported her moods, her wishes, her dreams, arguments with patients or with nurses, crying bouts, etc.

Demonstration of Relationship

The recordings were tabulated after the patient left hospital. The following hypothesis was formulated: there existed a demonstrable relationship between meetings with her mother and "real asthmatic attacks."

Table 1 demonstrates the probability of such a relationship. Statistically this table yields a χ^2 of 10 (8 when Yates's correction is applied), which is significant beyond the 1% level.

TABLE 1

Occurrence of asthma	Days with asthma	Days without asthma
—	15	70
Within 24 hours of being with mother	9 (60 %)	14 (20 %)
Not in contact with mother for preceding 24 hours	6 (40 %)	56 (80 %)

Additional Findings

(*a*) *Mother and home*. Within this relationship the following is worth emphasizing. The patient saw her mother twenty-three times during her stay in hospital; these meetings rarely took place in the hospital, as the patient was allowed out for separate afternoons and for whole week-ends, and could therefore meet her mother either at home or elsewhere. The twenty-three occasions when she saw her mother were divided into "with mother at home" and "with mother but outside home." Although here the χ^2 lies only between the 0.05 and 0.10 level of significance, Table 2

TABLE 2

	Followed by asthma	Not followed by asthma
Meeting mother at home	7	5
Meeting mother outside home	2	9

suggests that the situation 'mother-home' was more closely related to the attacks than the 'mother-out' one.

Three visits at home alone when the mother was absent did not result in any attack. Moreover, the patient spent two week-ends with friends in their homes again with no subsequent attacks.

(*b*) Other events, such as the occurrence of interviews, violent exercise (tennis, dancing) or marked changes in the weather, had been recorded. On inspection there did not emerge any relationship comparable to that demonstrated. Nor was there any indication of a temporal regularity which would have suggested a connexion between attacks and the patient's menstrual cycle.

(*c*) The value as a means of prediction of the relationship observed during her stay in hospital, was tested after her discharge. The attacks had by then become much less frequent. Before entering hospital the patient said she had suffered daily attacks during the preceding two years. For a week prior to, and for five days following, her admission she suffered no attack. Dividing the rest of her stay in hospital into two periods of 40 days, she experienced thirteen attacks during the first period and two attacks during the second period. After her discharge she periodically reported to the Out-patients Department and the occurrence of her attacks has been recorded, albeit in a much less reliable fashion for 20 months after her discharge. She was then living away from home in pleasant surroundings but went occasionally to see her mother in London. After a few months she married and, despite disagreement with her mother-in-law, the marriage proved happy and successful. She carried on with her job as a hairdresser in another branch of the same firm and in a much more congenial atmosphere.

During these 20 months she reported nine attacks, and the prediction that they would occur in conjunction with the "mother-home" situation was verified in eight out of nine cases.

DISCUSSION

This investigation shows the possibility of demonstrating objectively a connexion between a specific emotion (defined here as an environmental situation which is assumed to be emotionally loaded) and the occurrence of an asthmatic attack. Some aspects of this method of observation and demonstration require comment:

(*a*) The establishment of such a connexion in no way diminishes the importance of the constitutional predisposition, nor does it exclude the possibility of causation by physical stimuli. Moreover, although at this phase of the patient's life it is the mother who seems to be endowed with emotional significance and who thereby provokes attacks, it may nevertheless be that any emotion however caused—provided it reached a high enough intensity and mobilizing power—could have the same effect.

(*b*) Suggestion may well have played a part; the physician had told the patient at the beginning of her stay and twice again later that her mother was linked to her disturbance. This does not invalidate the demonstration of the connexion between the two events, but it does indicate the desirability of controlling the use of suggestion in future similar work.

(*c*) At the beginning of the investigation the patient had been presented with verbal and pictorial stimuli connected with her mother, but these did not provoke any attack. Nor was there any relationship between the many interviews at which she discussed her mother and an ensuing attack. This, together with Table 2, suggests that for this girl, the more concrete the situation, the more effective it is in its psychogenic causation. But further work may show that with a more intelligent, introspective and introverted subject, ideas or symbolic representation, much less amenable to objective recording, would play a larger part in the precipitation of the attacks.

SUMMARY

This report on an asthmatic patient demonstrates the existence of a significant relationship between her attacks and the emotional situation of meeting her mother. The conclusion is derived from the recording of as many observations as possible during her stay in hospital and holds true for a period of almost two years following her discharge.

REFERENCES

FRENCH, T. M. & ALEXANDER, F. (1941). Psychogenic factors in bronchial asthma. *Psychosom. Med. Monogr.* no. 4. National Research Council, Washington, D.C.

LEIGH, D. (1953). Asthma and the psychiatrist. A clinical review. *Int. Arch. Allergy, N.Y., 4,* 4, 227.

Part III

Applications in Treatment

A few illustrations of the use of experimental approaches in behavior modification are presented in the papers of Part III. We are reminded by the classical paper of Mary Cover Jones that such an approach is by no means new. Indeed, it is unfortunate that, although nearly half a century has passed since this study, the techniques of alleviating a patient's fears have improved so little.

The approach being advocated in this book is applicable to a wide variety of patient complaints as indicated in the contrast between the next two papers in this Part. On the one hand we have the treatment of a reading disability by Ancevich and Payne, and on the other hand, the treatment by Shapiro of a woman with phobic and depressive symptoms. The paper by Shapiro is of particular value in that it describes his Personal Questionnaire technique. This technique is particularly suited to the study of individual cases and once again demonstrates that one need not neglect the idiosyncrasies of a patient when experimentally investigating or treating his disorder.

The adoption of the experimental approach does not necessitate the abandoning of present methods of treatment. This is indicated in the paper by Murray in which he describes the content analysis of conventional psychotherapy sessions. As Murray notes, his paper ". . . demonstrates the applicability of principles derived from animal and human experimentation to complex human behavior." He goes on to say that such clarification of clinical data will stimulate experimental work and modify existing theories. These are important points and a two-way relationship between experimental and clinical psychology is absolutely necessary if the science of psychology is to progress.

One of the more important recent developments in clinical psychology has been the application of Skinner's theory of learning to the modification of patient behavior. An example of such application is given in the description by Tate and Baroff of the treatment of a nine-year-old blind psychotic boy.

In the early 1950's one of the most important developments in psychiatry occurred with the appearance of psychoactive drugs. The proper evaluation of the effects of these drugs has unfortunately not proceeded as well as one would have wished. This is partly due to the difficulty of doing group studies with drugs. It is for this reason that the demonstration in the last paper by Bellak and Chassan, of the application of single case experimentation to the study of the effects of a drug, is so important.

10

A Laboratory Study of Fear: The Case of Peter*

MARY COVER JONES

As part of a genetic study of emotions, a number of children were observed in order to determine the most effective methods of removing fear responses.

The case of Peter illustrates how a fear may be removed under laboratory conditions. His case was selected from a number of others for the following reasons:

1. Progress in combating the fear reactions was so marked that many of the details of the process could be observed easily.
2. It was possible to continue the study over a period of more than three months.
3. The notes of a running diary show the characteristics of a healthy, normal, interesting child, well adjusted, except for his exaggerated fear reactions. A few descriptive notes show something of his personality:

> Remarkably active, easily interested, capable of prolonged endeavor. . . . A favorite with the children as well as with the nurses and matrons . . . Peter has a healthy passion for possessions. Everything that he lays his hands on is his. As this is frequently disputed by some other child, there are occasional violent scenes of protest. These disturbances are not more frequent than might be expected in a three-year-old, in view of the fact that he is continually forced to adjust to a large group of children, nor are they more marked in Peter's case than in others of his age. Peter's I. Q. at the age of 2 years and 10 months was 102 on the Kuhlmann Revision of the Binet. At the same time he passed 5 of the 3 year tests on the Stan-

* Reprinted from *The Pedagogical Seminary and Journal of Genetic Psychology,* 1924, Vol. 31, pp. 308–315, by permission of the author and the publisher.

ford Revision. In initiative and constructive ability, however, he is superior to his companions of the same mental age.

4. This case is a sequel to one recently contributed by Dr. Watson and furnished supplementary material of interest in a genetic study of emotions. Dr. Watson's case illustrated how a fear could be produced experimentally under laboratory conditions. A brief review follows: Albert, eleven months of age, was an infant with a phlegmatic disposition, afraid of nothing "under the sun" except a loud sound made by striking a steel bar. This made him cry. By striking the bar at the same time that Albert touched a white rat, the fear was transferred to the white rat. After seven combined stimulations, rat and sound, Albert not only became greatly disturbed at the sight of a rat, but this fear had spread to include a white rabbit, cotton wool, a fur coat, and the experimenter's hair. It did not transfer to his wooden blocks and other objects very dissimilar to the rat.

In referring to this case, Dr. Watson says, "We have shown experimentally that when you condition a child to show fear of an animal, this fear transfers or spreads in such a way that without separate conditioning he becomes afraid of many animals. If you take any one of these objects producing fear and uncondition, will fear of the other objects in the series disappear at the same time? That is, will the unconditioning spread without further training to other stimuli?"

Dr. Watson intended to continue the study of Albert in an attempt to answer this question, but Albert was removed from the hospital and the series of observations was discontinued.

About three years later this case, which seemed almost to be Albert grown a bit older, was discovered in our laboratory.

Peter was 2 years and 10 months old when we began to study him. He was afraid of a white rat, and this fear extended to a rabbit, a fur coat, a feather, cotton wool, etc., but not to wooden blocks and similar toys. An abridgment of the first laboratory notes on Peter reads as follows:

Peter was put in a crib in a play room and immediately became absorbed in his toys. A white rat was introduced into the crib from behind. (The etxperimenter was behind a screen). At sight of the rat, Peter screamed and fell flat on his back in a paroxysm of fear. The stimulus was removed, and Peter was taken out of the crib and put into a chair. Barbara was brought to the crib and the white rat introduced as before. She exhibited no fear but picked the rat up in her hand. Peter sat quietly watching Barbara and the rat. A string of beads belonging to Peter had been left in the crib. Whenever the rat touched a part of the string he would say "my beads" in a complaining voice, although he made no objections when Barbara touched them. Invited to get down from the chair, he shook his head, fear not yet subsided. Twenty-five minutes elapsed before he was ready to play about freely.

The next day his reactions to the following situations and objects were noted:

Play room and crib	Selected toys, got into crib without protest
White ball rolled in	Picked it up and held it
Fur rug hung over crib	Cried until it was removed
Fur coat hung over crib	Cried until it was removed
Cotton	Whimpered, withdrew, cried
Hat with feathers	Cried
Blue woolly sweater	Looked, turned away, no fear
White toy rabbit of rough cloth	No interest, no fear
Wooden doll	No interest, no fear

This case made it possible for the experiment to continue where Dr. Watson had left off. The first problem was that of "unconditioning" a fear response to an animal, and the second, that of determining whether unconditioning to one stimulus spreads without further training to other stimuli.

From the test situations which were used to reveal fears, it was found that Peter showed even more marked fear responses to the rabbit than to the rat. It was decided to use the rabbit for unconditioning and to proceed as follows: Each day Peter and three other children were brought to the laboratory for a play period. The other children were selected carefully because of their entirely fearless attitude toward the rabbit and because of their satisfactory adjustments in general. The rabbit was always present during a part of the play period. From time to time Peter was brought in alone so that his reactions could be observed and progress noted.

From reading over the notes for each session it was apparent that there had been improvement by more or less regular steps from almost complete terror at sight of the rabbit to a completely positive response with no signs of disturbance. New situations requiring closer contact with the rabbit had been gradually introduced and the degree to which these situations were avoided, tolerated, or welcomed, at each experimental session, gave the measure of improvement. Analysis of the notes on Peter's reactions indicated the following progressive steps in his degrees of toleration:

A. Rabbit anywhere in the room in a cage causes fear reactions.

B. " 12 feet away in cage tolerated.

C. " 4 " " " " "

D. " 3 " " " " "

E. " close in cage tolerated.

F. " free in room tolerated.

G. " touched when experimenter holds it.

H. " touched when free in room.

I. " defied by spitting at it, throwing things at it, imitating it.

J. " allowed on tray of high chair.

K. Squats in defenseless position beside rabbit.

L. Helps experimenter to carry rabbit to its cage.

M. Holds rabbit on lap.

N. Stays alone in room with rabbit.

O. Allows rabbit in play pen with him.

P. Fondles rabbit affectionately.

Q. Lets rabbit nibble his fingers.

These "degrees of toleration" merely represented the stages in which improvement occurred. They did not give any indications of the intervals between steps, nor of the plateaus, relapses, and sudden gains which were actually evident. To show these features a curve was drawn by using the seventeen steps given above as the Y axis of a chart and the experimental sessions as the X axis. The units are not equal on either axis, as the "degrees of toleration" have merely been set down as they appeared from consideration of the laboratory notes with no attempt to evaluate the steps. Likewise the experimental sessions were not equi-distant in time. Peter was seen twice daily for a period and thence only once a day. At one point illness and quarantine interrupted the experiments for two months. There is no indication of these irregularities on the chart. For example, along the X axis, 1 represents the date December 4th when the observation began. 11 and 12 represent the dates March 10 A.M. and P.M. (from December 17 to March 7, Peter was not available for study).

The question arose as to whether or not the points on the Y axis which indicated progress to the experimenter represented

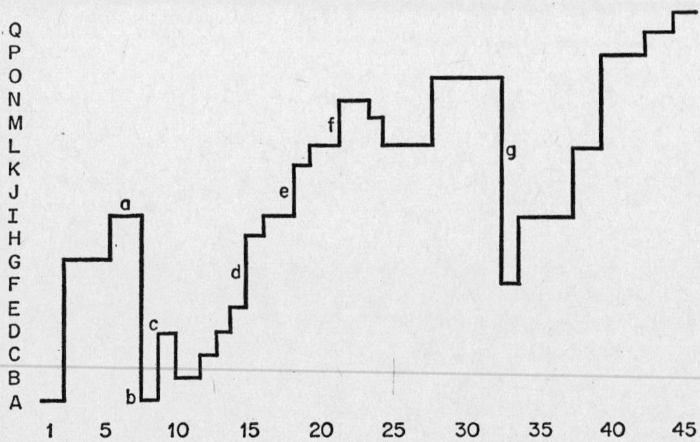

real advance and not merely idiosyncratic reactions of the subject. The "tolerance series" as indicated by the experimenter was presented in random order to six graduate students and instructors in psychology to be arranged so as to indicate increase in tolerance, in their judgment. An average correlation of .70 with the experimenter's arrangement was found for the six ratings. This indicates that the experimenter was justified from an a priori point of view in designating the steps to be progressive stages.

The first seven periods show how Peter progressed from a great fear of the rabbit to a tranquil indifference and even a voluntary pat on the rabbit's back when others were setting the example. The notes for the seventh period (see a on chart) read:

Laurel, Mary, Arthur, Peter playing together in the laboratory. Experimenter put rabbit down on floor. Arthur said, "Peter doesn't cry when he sees the rabbit come out." Peter, "No." He was a little concerned as to whether or not the rabbit would eat his kiddie car. Laurel and Mary stroked the rabbit and chattered away excitedly. Peter walked over, touched the rabbit on the back, exulting, "I touched him on the end."

At this period Peter was taken to the hospital with scarlet fever. He did not return for two months.

By referring to the chart at (b), it will be noted that the line shows a decided drop to the early level of fear reaction when he returned. This was easily explained by the nurse who brought Peter from the hospital. As they were entering a taxi at the door of the hospital, a large dog, running past, jumped at them. Both Peter and the nurse were very much frightened, Peter so much that he lay back in the taxi pale and quiet, and the nurse debated whether or not to return him to the hospital. This seemed reason enough for his precipitate descent back to the original fear level. Being threatened by a large dog when ill, and in a strange place and being with an adult who also showed fear, was a terrifying situation against which our training could not have fortified him.

At this point (b) we began another method of treatment, that of "direct conditioning." Peter was seated in a high chair and given food which he liked. The experimenter brought the rabbit in a wire cage as close as she could without arousing a response which would interfere with the eating. Through the presence of the pleasant stimulus (food) whenever the rabbit was shown, the fear was eliminated gradually in favor of a positive response. Occasionally also, other children were brought in to help with the "unconditioning." These facts are of interest in following the charted progress. The first decided rise at (c) was due to the presence of another child who influenced Peter's reaction. The notes for this day read:

Lawrence and Peter sitting near together in their high chairs eating candy. Rabbit in cage put down 12 feet away. Peter began to cry. Lawrence said, "Oh, rabbit." Clambered down, ran over and looked in the cage at him. Peter followed close and watched.

The next two decided rises at (d) and (e) occurred on the day when a student assistant, Dr. S., was present. Peter was very fond of Dr. S. whom he insisted was his "papa." Although Dr. S. did not directly influence Peter by any overt suggestions, it may be that having him there contributed to Peter's general feeling of well being and thus indirectly affected his reactions. The fourth rise on the chart at (f) was, like the first, due to the influence of another child. Notes for the 21st session read:

> Peter with candy in high chair. Experimenter brought rabbit and sat down in front of the tray with it. Peter cried out, "I don't want him," and withdrew. Rabbit was given to another child sitting near to hold. His holding the rabbit served as a powerful suggestion; Peter wanted the rabbit on his lap, and held it for an instant.

The decided drop at (g) was caused by a slight scratch when Peter was helping to carry the rabbit to his cage. The rapid ascent following shows how quickly he regained lost ground.

In one of our last sessions, Peter showed no fear although another child was present who showed marked disturbance at sight of the rabbit.

An attempt was made from time to time to see what verbal organization accompanied this process of "unconditioning." Upon Peter's return from the hospital, the following conversation took place:

> E.: (experimenter) What do you do upstairs, Peter? (The laboratory was upstairs).
> P.: I see my brother. Take me up to see my brother.
> E.: What else will you see?
> P.: Blocks.

Peter's reference to blocks indicated a definite memory as he played with blocks only in the laboratory. No further response of any significance could be elicited. In the laboratory two days later (he had seen the rabbit once in the meantime), he said suddenly, "Beads can't bite me, beads can only look at me." Toward the end of the training an occasional "I like the rabbit," was all the language he had to parallel the changed emotional organization.

Early in the experiment an attempt was made to get some measure of the visceral changes accompanying Peter's fear reactions. On one occasion Dr. S. determined Peter's blood pressure outside the laboratory and again later, in the laboratory while he was in a state of much anxiety caused by the rabbit's being held close to him by the experimenter. The diastolic blood pressure changed from 65 to 80 on this occasion. Peter was taken to the infirmary the next day for the routine physical examination and developed there a suspicion of medical instruments which made it inadvisable to proceed with this phase of the work.

Peter has gone home to a difficult environment but the experimenter is still in touch with him. He showed in the last interview, as on the later portions of the chart, a genuine fondness for the rabbit. What has happened to the fear of the other objects? The fear of the cotton, the fur coat, feathers, was entirely absent at our last interview. He looked at them, handled them, and immediately turned to something which interested him more. The reaction to the rats, and the fur rug with the stuffed head was greatly modified and improved. While he did not show the fondness for these that was apparent with the rabbit, he had made a fair adjustment. For example, Peter would pick up the tin box containing frogs or rats and carry it around the room. When requested, he picked up the fur rug and carried it to the experimenter.

What would Peter do if confronted by a strange animal? At the last interview the experimenter presented a mouse and a tangled mass of angleworms. At first sight, Peter showed slight distress reactions and moved away, but before the period was over he was carrying the worms about and watching the mouse with undisturbed interest. By "unconditioning" Peter to the rabbit, he has apparently been helped to overcome many superfluous fears, some completely, some to a less degree. His tolerance of strange animals and unfamiliar situations has apparently increased.

The study is still incomplete. Peter's fear of the animals which were shown him was probably not a directly conditioned fear. It is unlikely that he had ever had any experience with white rats, for example. Where the fear originated and with what stimulus, is not known. Nor is it known what Peter would do if he were again confronted with the original fear situation. All of the fears which were "unconditioned" were transferred fears, and it has not yet been learned whether or not the primary fear can be eliminated by training the transfers.

Another matter which must be left to speculation is the future welfare of the subject. His "home" consists of one furnished room which is occupied by his mother and father, a brother of nine years and himself. Since the death of an older sister, he is the recipient of most of the unwise affection of his parents. His brother appears to bear him a grudge because of this favoritism, as might be expected. Peter hears continually, "Ben is so bad and so dumb, but Peter is so good and so smart!" His mother is a highly emotional individual who can not get through an interview, however brief, without a display of tears. She is totally incapable of providing a home on the $25 a week which her husband steadily earns. In an attempt to control Peter she resorts to frequent fear suggestions. "Come in, Peter, some one wants to steal you." To her erratic resorts to discipline, Peter reacts with temper tantrums. He was denied a summer in the country because his father "forgets he's tired when he has Peter around." Surely a discouraging outlook for Peter.

But the recent development of psychological studies of young children and the growing tendency to carry the knowledge gained in the psychological laboratories into the home and school induce us to predict a more wholesome treatment of a future generation of Peters.

11

The Investigation and Treatment of a Reading Disability in a Child of Normal Intelligence*

Singrida S. Ancevich and R. W. Payne

CASE REPORT

This paper describes an experimental investigation of a nine-year-old boy, Harry, who was backward at school, with severe difficulties in reading, writing and spelling. He was also a mild behavior problem, and was an out-patient at the Mental Health Clinic, Kingston, during this investigation.

Family History

Harry's parents are first cousins, a fact which has always caused great anxiety to his mother. For about four and a half years the marriage was happy, although the father changed jobs frequently. However when Harry's older brother, who is now twelve, was one year of age, the father left to take up a job as a bricklayer in the United States. He returned for a few hours when Harry was a week and a half old, intimated to the mother that the child was not his, was very evasive about his plans, and disappeared. He has not been seen since, and the children have been told he is dead. The mother at present appears lonely and depressed, and believes that her main problem is the lack of a father in the house.

The mother has been wearing a hearing aid for over fifteen years. Her brother is deaf as well, and her sister became completely deaf at age 17. She reports that both boys have poor academic habits, and frequently quarrel. Although the older boy

* Reprinted from the *Journal of Clinical Psychology,* 1961, Vol. 17, pp. 416–420, by permission of the authors and the publisher.

performs well academically, both boys are frequently disobedient and impudent. The mother says she occasionally slaps the face of the offender, although she reported that she uses no other corporal punishment.

Personal History

Harry is the younger of two brothers by three years. He was a full term baby, although the membranes ruptured four weeks before birth. He walked at 15 months, but did not talk until over two. This was probably due to the fact that he was "tongue-tied" from birth. At three he underwent an operation which cut the thread connecting the tongue. He still has some difficulty with his speech which has a nasal sound.

Harry was also born with a deformed right ear. At the age of one he had earaches due to an abundance of wax. An operation to correct the external deformity was performed at the age of six, although it was only partly successful. Harry still complains periodically of a buzzing sound in this ear, and an occasional difficulty with hearing which disappears, he says, if he bangs his head several times. He has been taken frequently to a physician about the ear, who reports that his hearing is now normal. However, in the clinic it was noted that his speech has a nasal sound, and he appears to have difficulty in pronouncing some sounds (the letter "t", "th" and "s").

Harry is backward scholastically. He repeated grade two, and he was only in grade three when first seen, at the age of nine years and five months among children whose average age is eight. He was referred by his mother to the Mental Health Clinic with the following complaints: (a) He daydreams, (b) talks to himself, (c) is unwilling to do things, (d) dislikes reading and writing, and (e) never finishes anything at school. The mother especially complained that Harry always voiced resentment when she told him about his scholastic backwardness.

PSYCHOLOGICAL STUDIES

The psychologist was asked to explain Harry's backwardness in reading which had not responded to extra coaching in school. Harry was given the Wechsler Intelligence Scale for Children when he first came to the clinic. His scores were: Full Scale IQ 95; Verbal IQ 90; Performance IQ 101. The tests were consistent in suggesting an average intellectual ability, and that his reading disability was not the result of defective intelligence.

The first hypothesis put forward was that Harry's reading backwardness was the result of a partial hearing loss. It was noted that Harry seldom pronounced the letter "t" when it occurred at the end of a word, as in "raft" or "lost." He also pronounced "s" almost as "sh" except where it occurred at the beginning of a word. Frequently he could not pronounce "th". It was speculated that high frequency deafness may have impaired word perception, which made the association of letters and sounds difficult, and which also affected his pronunciation. Harry was referred for an audiometric examination by a medical specialist, who again reported normal hearing. It was then concluded that this speech was the result of the early tongue deformity noted above, and was not connected with his reading difficulty.

In order to investigate his reading difficulty further, Harry was given the Durrell (1955) Analysis of Reading Difficulties. The results were:

Reading	
Oral reading	Grade 3.0 level
Silent reading	Grade 3.0 level
Comprehension	Grade 4.0 level
Word recognition	below Grade 2 level (score = 0)
Word analysis	Grade 3.0 level
Letters	
Naming letters	
Identifying letters named	no errors
Matching letters	
Visual Memory of Words	Grade 2.5 level
Sounds	
Hearing sounds in words	Grade 3.5 level
Hearing sounds in letters	Grade 3.5 level
Learning to hear sounds in words	no errors
Spelling	
Phonic spelling of words	Score 0
Spelling test	Grade 2.5 level
Handwriting: Speed	Below Grade 2 level—19 words per minute

These results suggested the following tentative conclusions: (a) Harry's oral and silent reading ability were at the grade 3 level, exactly consistent with his school grade, but one year backward for children of his age. This performance was slightly better than one would have expected from his mother's complaints. It was not possible to say how frequently a discrepancy of this magnitude would occur, between the average WISC IQ and the reading ability on this test, because of lack of data about the two tests concerned. (b) Harry's ability to perform a phonic analysis of words was consistent with his general level of reading. (c) His reading comprehension was exactly average for his age, in spite of his reading backwardness, and consistent with his average intelligence. (d) There was no evidence of a perceptual difficulty in connection with reading. He was well able to discriminate between, and name individual letters. (e) There was no evidence for a learning failure in the auditory modality. Harry was able to associate sounds with individual letters, and with words at an average level for his age. (d) His main abnormality was his inability to recognize and remember whole words presented visually. His visual memory for words was only at the grade 2.5 level, and his tachistoscopic recognition of words was below the grade 2 level (he recognized no words at all presented in this way). His score on a written spelling test was also at the grade 2.5 level, while on an oral spelling test he did even worse, getting no words correct. His handwriting speed was very slow, again below the grade 2 level.

These findings suggested that a possible explanation for his reading backwardness was that he had a specific learning defect, being unable to learn associations in the visual modality. Such relatively specific learning abnormalities have been reported (*1*) before, in children who are backward readers. If this were the case, it was thought that a program of special coaching, emphasizing the formation of connections in the auditory modality, in which he was apparently normal, would be effective.

It was intended to test this hypothesis further, by means of a learning experiment, investigating the patient's ability for paired associate learning in all modalities. Before this experiment was carried out however, a further observation was made which suggested an alternative hypothesis. It was noticed that Harry was left handed, but that he had been taught to write with his paper slanted towards the left, like a right handed pupil. When he wrote in this way, he covered from view the letters and words which he had already written, only the last letter being visible to him at any given time. It was thought that this might seriously impair his learning, since he never saw a complete word when writing himself, and would thus have very much less practice in learning to recognize whole words. Indeed, writing, for him, was a series of discrete letters. It was thought that this very simple fact could explain his almost complete failure to learn to spell, and his difficulty in recognizing whole words tachistoscopically (but his ability to piece them together letter by letter, phonetically). This could also explain his slowness in reading and writing.

INVESTIGATION OF THE HYPOTHESIS

To test this hypothesis, three equivalent groups of 15 words each were selected. The first group was the first fifteen words which Harry could not spell from the Mill Hill Vocabulary Scale, Form 1, Junior (*3*). The second group was the first fifteen words which he could not spell from the Mill Hill Vocabulary Form 2, Junior, and the third group was the first fifteen words he could not spell from the Stanford Binet Vocabulary Scale (*4*). The lists used are presented in Table 1.

Procedure

Each word was printed on a card which fitted into a cardboard case. The words were presented to Harry tachistoscopically for half a second by flashing a shutter, according to the method of tachistoscopic presentation used in the Durrell (*2*) Analysis of Reading Difficulty. After a word was flashed, Harry was asked to write down what he had seen. Harry made no correct response with Group 1 words, and only one with Groups 2 and 3. For all practical purposes the groups were identical, in that the patient was unable to recognize the words in any of the groups when they were presented tachistoscopically.

Harry was then taught to spell each list of words. He was taught list 1 by showing him each word (which was printed on

TABLE 1

The Three Groups of Words Selected for Presentation

Group 1	Group 2	Group 3
loaf	tomato	orange
disturb	rest	envelope
battle	patch	straw
receive	afraid	puddle
view	cruel	game
continue	blaze	eyelash
startle	ache	roar
perfume	squabble	scorch
malaria	rage	muzzle
mingle	shrivel	haste
fascinated	connect	lecture
prosper	provide	skill
anonymous	stubborn	juggle
verify	schooner	brunette
ruse	liberty	peculiarity

an individual card) tachistoscopically according to the method of administration used in the Durrell (*2*) test. He was then asked to write it down. The words were presented in order until the criterion of three consecutive correct spellings of each word was achieved. When the criterion was reached for a word, that word was dropped from the list.

For list 2, the patient was given a large square card with a small square hole cut in the middle of it. The administration was identical with the administration used for list 1, except that when writing down each word, Harry was asked to put this card on the paper, and to write each letter through the hole, moving it up for each letter so that the last letter written was completely covered. It was predicted that the results would be the same as for list 1, since Harry's normal method of writing obscured what he had written, much like the shield.

For list 3, the same method of administration was followed, excepting that this time Harry was made to write so that he could see all he had written. Before this part of the experiment was performed, he was trained for a week to write with his paper slanted to the right rather than to the left, and to slant his handwriting to the right by writing "backhand." In this way he could write a whole line without covering any of the words. This training required five sessions with the psychologist, during which

Harry was given simple practice exercises in writing. His teacher was told about this procedure, and she also encouraged Harry to use this new method at school. After a week of this instruction, Harry was taught the third list of words.

Results

The score for each condition was the total number of incorrect responses before the required criterion of three consecutive correct responses was reached. The results are presented in Table 2. Analysis of variance was used to assess the significance between

TABLE 2

Number of Trials Needed to Learn to Spell New Words

Condition	Mean	SD	F	*P*
Ordinary	6.066	6.69	4.95	<.01
Covered	6.53	6.73		
New	0.80	1.42		

the number of trials required for each condition. The results are significant at the .01 level, and support the hypothesis. Almost no difference was obtained between the number of trials required to reach the criterion under Harry's original way of writing, and when he wrote through a mask which covered every letter from view. Yet the number of trials required after Harry was taught to write in such a way that the letters were not covered, was remarkably smaller.

A few days later, the three groups of words were again presented tachistoscopically for half a second to determine to what extent this training now enabled Harry to read the words when presented tachistoscopically. Harry now correctly read 5, 10 and 7 words on lists 1, 2 and 3, as compared with 0, 1 and 1 words before training. The results suggested that Harry was better able to read these words after having been taught to spell them in this way, and that even although list 3 was learned much more quickly, it was retained approximately as well as the other two lists.

It was concluded from these results that the hypothesized explanation of Harry's failure to learn to read was supported. Harry was, therefore, merely supervised at school to make sure he continued to write in the way he had been taught. He was given a small amount of extra attention by his school teacher, but no further coaching by the psychologist.

Six weeks after the experiment had been completed Harry was retested on the Durrell test with results shown in Table 3. Improvement is only shown on three of the five tests. We cannot be certain that this change represents a measureable finding, and is not within the range of error of measurement of the tests concerned (data are not available). Nevertheless the results are in the expected direction, and six weeks is a very short period in

TABLE 3

Grade Levels Achieved on the Durrell Analysis of Reading Difficulty before and after Instruction in New Method of Writing

	Reading Oral	Reading Silent	Word Recognition	Word Analysis	Spelling	Handwriting
Before	3.0	3.0	Below Grade 2 Score = 0	3.5	2.5	Below Grade 2
After	3.0	3.0	3.5	4.0	3.0	Below Grade 2

which to expect a dramatic improvement. The "handwriting" results are, for example, due to the fact that Harry was taught no further writing during this period, as his teacher still requires her pupils to print. The teacher did report that she thought that Harry's spelling had improved a great deal, and that his work was both neater and of a higher standard. Both the teacher and Harry's mother agreed that he was now more interested in his school work.

SUMMARY AND CONCLUSIONS

An experimental investigation was conducted with a boy of nine years, five months, who had difficulty in writing and spelling, and was unwilling to cooperate at school or do schoolwork at home. He was in Grade 3, one year retarded for his age, but his spelling and writing were below even Grade 3 level.

Since the child was left-handed, it was noticed that he covered each letter from view when constructing a word. It was hypothesized that, if he were trained to write in such a way that his letters would not be covered from view, he would form visual associations of sounds and words more quickly, and would improve in word recognition and hence spelling. Experiments supported the hypothesis. It required significantly fewer trials to obtain the criterion of three consecutive correct responses of words presented after the boy was given instruction in a new method of writing.

On retesting on an achievement test 6 weeks after the new method of writing had been taught, the results were in the predicted direction. His spelling and word recognition were now at the Grade 3 level. The teacher also reported that the boy's work was now much neater and that his writing and dictation had improved. He also seemed more willing to do his work.

REFERENCES

1. Bartlett, D. and Shapiro, M. B. Investigation and treatment of a reading disability in a dull child with severe psychiatric disturbances. *Brit. J. educat. Psychol.*, 1956, *26,* 180–190.
2. Durrell, D. D. *Manual for the Durrell Analysis of Reading Difficulty*. (New Revision) New York: Psychol. Corp., 1955.
3. Raven, J. C. *Guide to using the Mill Hill Vocabulary Scale with the Progressive Matrices Scale*. London: H. K. Lewis, 1958.
4. Terman, L. M. and Merrill, M. A. *Measuring Intelligence*. Cambridge, Mass.: Houghton Mifflin, 1937.

12

The Measurement of Clinically Relevant Variables*

M. B. SHAPIRO

The work reported in this paper is based upon two essential distinctions, both of which were made by Claude Bernard as early as 1865. The first distinction is that between observational and experimental research. In observational research the experimenter observes what nature presents to him, and tries to make his observations as reproducible as possible. In experimental research the observer systematically interferes with nature. He tries to manipulate it and bring it under some kind of control. Claude Bernard regarded this form of research as creative, as bringing to light important phenomena which otherwise remain unobserved.

The second distinction is between group centred and individual centred research. In group centred research the observations taken from the number of individuals are averaged. Claude Bernard pointed out that biological processes only take place in individual organisms and therefore could only be observed in individual organisms. Experimental psychology, except for the work of Skinner and his followers, has depended mainly upon group centred observations, for example, the growth of intelligence. In fact, there is evidence that growth curves of intelligence are, in terms of relative status to others of the same age, not the same for different individuals over a period of years. Goodenough (1946) quotes a study by Bailey demonstrating this point. Over a period of nine years, some subjects maintained average status throughout the period; some steadily lost status as they grew older; some did exactly the opposite, steadily im-

* Reprinted from the *Journal of Psychosomatic Research,* 1964, Vol. 8, pp. 245–254, by permission of the author and the publisher.

proving their status; a fourth group of subjects lost status at first and then regained it; a fifth group did the opposite, starting with a gain in status and then losing it. Finally, there were some subjects who provided no identifiable curves whatever. If this picture is correct, then the average negatively accelerated growth curve of intelligence has no existence in nature, and there is no point in investigating it. A similar argument applies to all psychological processes. It would seem to be sensible to combine data obtained from a number of individual subjects only when it has been demonstrated that the process under investigation behaves in the same way for all the individuals concerned.

There is a complete absence, in clinical psychology, of research which is based upon the psychological manipulation of psychological dysfunctions in individual patients. An attempt is now being made to deal with this problem (Shapiro, 1961b; Shapiro, 1963). The research to be reported in this paper marks the beginnings of an attempt to meet this need. Because our resources for research are extremely limited, we have had to restrict the scope of our work. First of all we have centred on one manifestation of psychological disorder: the patient's own assessment of it. We have not tried to deal with the two other important aspects: assessment by others and the directly measurable behaviour of the patient himself.

Our second restriction is in the method of measuring self-assessment. We have centred on the questionnaire because it is technically the least expensive and time-consuming, and because there is now a large experimental literature on the technical snags in the questionnaire. This knowledge enables us to take steps to minimise the influence of artefacts upon, and to maximise the reliability of, the patient's responses.

There are three main technical problems to be considered when devising questionnaires. The first is that of "irrelevant response set." This phrase refers to the fact that the response of the subject to a questionnaire is influenced by the form of presentation of the items as well as their content. (Christie *et al.*, 1958; Cronbach, 1950). For example, in many questionnaires each item is answered by pencilling a mark against "Yes," "?," or "No." It has been abundantly shown that some subjects have a consistent tendency to answer "Yes," some "?," and some "No," quite independently of the content of the items. Such tendencies can be demonstrated by giving the same group of subjects two questionnaires with contents of opposite directions. For example, in one study, all the statements in one questionnaire were drafted in such a way as to make all the "Yes" answerers agree to statements with a radical social content, and in the other questionnaire so as to make all the "Yes" answerers agree to statements with a conservative social content. The correlation between the two kinds of questionnaire was not highly negative, as would naively be expected, and in one study the correlation was actually slightly positive. Another example of a form of questionnaire which produces an irrelevant response set is one in which the subject is asked to indicate which of a number of items apply to him. Subjects will vary consistently in the proportion of items they will select, independently of the content.

It follows from these considerations that any kind of questionnaire technique must be as free as possible from any kind of form which is additional to the content. To coin a phrase, questionnaires have to be "form-free."

The second problem is that of the ambiguity of the content of the questionnaire items. Landis and Katz (1934) reported, some time ago, evidence that subjects often differed in their answers to the items of the questionnaire when in fact their "real" answers were the same, and *vice versa*. One example they gave is of an item which was concerned with fear of being in strange company. Some subjects selected "Yes" as an answer because, though they usually ended up by feeling comfortable, they always started by feeling anxious. A second group of subjects chose the "?," because they felt anxious to begin with and felt comfortable at the end. A third group chose "No" because, though they felt anxious to begin with, they always ended up by feeling comfortable. It is quite clear that it is necessary to have a technique which ensures that the subject understands the content of the questionnaire.

The third problem is that of reliability, in the sense of consistency of response. In the first place one needs a form of questionnaire which maximises the consistency of a subject's responses. This occurs when the subject only has to make a choice between two items at a time (Fiske, 1957). In the second place one needs to have an indication of the reliability or consistency of a given test result.

MEASURING THE DEPENDENT VARIABLE

The particular method we have developed is called the "Personal Questionnaire" (Shapiro, 1961a; Shapiro, 1961c). The development of this technique has been contributed to by many people, chief among whom were Mrs. B. Fox and Dr. F. Post. A special questionnaire is constructed for each subject, and it takes an experienced psychologist about four hours work to do so with the help of about two hours work from a typist. There are five phases in the construction of this questionnaire.

The first phase consists of a controlled interview in which all the possible introductory questions have been written out, and in which the general aims and methods of enquiry are defined. By the end of the interview, the psychologist has recorded a number of statements, each of which describes one of the patient's symptoms in his own words. Table 1 gives an example of such a test.

In the second phase the psychologist shows his list to the patient's psychiatrist. If there is any disagreement about the presence and absence of symptoms, they interview the patient together. This is rarely necessary.

The third phase consists of the construction, by the psychologist, of further statements which describe each symptom in varying degrees of improvement up to recovery. We have begun to devise rules of constructing these statements to speed up the procedure. At the moment, for reasons of convenience, we construct only three statements per symptom. One statement expresses a sufficient degree of unpleasantness of experience to warrant, in the judgment of the clinicians concerned, immediate treatment. A second statement indicates some improvement, and a third implies a sufficient absence of unpleasantness of experience to warrant the cessation of treatment (See Table 2 for examples). Thus, if there were originally statements describing 30 symptoms, there would now be 90 statements. As far as possible, the patient's initial formulations are preserved when writing these statements.

The fourth phase consists of the calibration of each statement by the patient himself. He does this in terms of the implications of unpleasantness of experience, which each statement has for

TABLE 1

Statement of Symptoms

1. It is very difficult for me to think of what I want when I go shopping.
2. When I'm in a shop I often feel I want to run out.
3. I find it very difficult to find the courage to start my daily walks.
4. I feel I cannot go into the garden by myself.
5. I don't like meeting people because I'm lost for words.
6. I have a fear I may fall down.
7. I am worried constantly about what effect my state will have on my daughter.
8. I feel inadequate as a mother.
9. I feel like a child.
10. I certainly feel my eyes will give out.
11. I am afraid I may forget who I am.
12. My legs feel like jelly.
13. I get a funny feeling so that I can't think of what I'm doing.
14. I feel no use at all.
15. My worries are part of me so that I can't get rid of them.
16. I feel conscious of my heart's action.
17. I certainly have a funny feeling in my head and want to poke my fingers into my ears to remove it.
18. I certainly feel my tummy turning over.
19. Everything around me seems real and I'm not.
20. I feel guilty about everything.
21. I have lost interest in everything.
22. I feel exhausted.
23. I feel I've been ill for so long I haven't got a future.

him. For this purpose a card is placed in front of the patient, and on it are written a list of nine hedonic phrases (See Table 3). Each statement is placed before the patient, one at a time, and he is asked to say which of the nine phrases best describes the hedonic implications of the statement before him. We want

TABLE 2

Examples of Questionnaire Statements

(i)	On the whole I have some energy.	Recovery.
(ii)	I have a little energy.	Improvement.
(iii)	I have not got any energy.	Illness.
(i)	On the whole I do not feel I look peculiar.	Recovery.
(ii)	I feel it is possible I look peculiar.	Improvement.
(iii)	I feel certain I look peculiar.	Illness.

TABLE 3

List of Hedonic Phrases

Very great pleasure
Very pleasant
Moderately pleasant
Slightly pleasant
Indifferent
Slightly unpleasant
Moderately unpleasant
Very unpleasant
Very great displeasure

each kind of statement to have roughly the same implications of unpleasantness. We aim to have all the illness statements rated by the patient as having implications which are very unpleasant or very greatly unpleasant, all the improvement statements as having moderately or slightly unpleasant implications, and all the recovery statements as having slightly or moderately pleasant implications. An additional aim of this method is that it might help to ensure comparability of changes in different symptoms.

If the patient does not rate a statement in the intended manner, then we obtain his cooperation in arriving at a reformulation which he in fact would accept at the intended level. This procedure has the incidental effect of helping to ensure that the patient has the same understanding of the questionnaire as the psychologist. Table 2 gives examples of two sets of such statements.

The fifth stage consists of the preparation of material for the actual test which will be administered to the patient. The form of the test is that of pair comparisons. This form provides (Shapiro, 1961a) a means of: (i) minimising the influence of irrelevant response sets (ii) maximising the reliability of test responses and (iii) providing some indication of reliability. Each pair of statements is typed on a separate card. There are thus three cards for each symptom. If there were originally 30 symptoms there would be 90 cards. In the actual test the patient is presented with one card at a time, in random order. He is instructed to indicate which of any given pair of statements is closer to his actual state at the time of doing the test (See Table 4).

TABLE 4

Examples of an Arrangement for Pair Comparisons

(iii) I have not got any energy.
(ii) I have a little energy.

(ii) I have a little energy.
(i) On the whole I have some energy.

(i) On the whole I have some energy.
(iii) I have not got any energy.

The scoring of the responses rests upon the fact that there are, in our material, eight different patterns of response (see Table 5). If the patient were ill in relation to a particular symptom, he would prefer statement (iii) to statements (i) and (ii), and statement (ii) to statement (i). This set of responses would constitute what we call a response pattern (No. IV in Table 5). If

TABLE 5

Showing Response Patterns

No.			
I	i →– ii	i →– iii	ii →– iii
II	i –← ii	i →– iii	ii →– iii
III	i –← ii	i –← iii	ii →– iii
IV	i –← ii	i –← iii	ii –← iii
V	i →– ii	i –← iii	ii →– iii
VI	i –← ii	i →– iii	ii –← iii
VII	i →– ii	i →– iii	ii –← iii
VIII	i –← ii	i –← iii	ii →– iii

i = recovery statements
ii = improvement statements
iii = illness statements
→– = prefer to e.g. i →– ii = i preferred to ii
i –← ii = ii preferred to i

the patient were improving he would prefer statement (ii) to statements (iii) and (i), the degree of improvement being indicated by his choice between statements (i) and (iii) (Nos. II and III in Table 5). If the patient were recovered he would prefer statement (i) to (iii) and (ii), and statement (ii) to (iii) (No. I in Table 5). There are four other response-patterns which would be produced if the patient were not responding consistently to the questionnaire. The proportion of these give an indication of the consistency of the patient's response to the questionnaire. Here we have some kind of measure of reliability.

Each of these five phases of the construction of the personal questionnaire presents problems which require further research. An attempt will now be made to give some concrete indication of how the personal questionnaire might be used to carry out research into the psychological disorders of psychiatric patients.

MANIPULATING THE INDEPENDENT VARIABLE

Two points must be made about this kind of research. In the first place, it is not possible to enter into a long term relationship with a patient, purely upon the basis of his serving as an experimental subject, when the intention is that of experimenting with his illness. It is impossible to treat another person as a mere guinea pig, when important and distressing aspects of his experience are being dealt with. This means that clinically relevant experimentation must, in the first place, be therapeutic in aim. The primary purpose must be to do all in one's power to help the patient concerned. The first decision, in this kind of experiment, is to decide first what one would try to do to help the patient, and having decided upon this, to ask oneself what kind of experiment was possible within the framework of the decisions taken.

The second point is that we decided to concentrate our research upon patients for whom the prognosis for any available treatment appeared to be bad. We wanted to learn more about the psychological processes occurring in such illnesses. We therefore chose to work on chronic depression. My colleagues and I have so far had experience of one short-term and two long-term experiments of this kind. We have so far only published the results of the short term experiment (Shapiro, Marks and Fox, 1963) and it is this experiment which we will outline briefly here. The experiment was carried out upon a 38 year old woman, with phobic and depressive symptoms of many years standing, who had been under various forms of treatment for the previous months. The illness statements which were used in the Personal Questionnaire are shown in Table 1. The independent variable was that of psychological treatment. This was varied in two ways: (i) by the application of a form of non-directive psychotherapy by the psychiatrist Dr. I. Marks, and (ii) by the application by the psychologists of a form of what might be called rational training, i.e. a mixture of behaviour therapy and rational psychotherapy. The two forms of treatment had been decided upon on purely clinical grounds. It was only subsequently that the experiment was devised. In the non-directive psychotherapy the patient was encouraged to express aggressive and sexual feelings. In the rational training treatment, the patient's feelings of guilt about being ill were modified by rational discussion, and her agoraphobia was treated by a method of desensitisation derived from Jones (1956). This consisted of walking increasingly long distances in the company of the therapists.

Figure 1 presents the design of the experiment. It was carried out over a period of four weeks with four treatments per week. Each kind of treatment was carried out in blocks of two, with a questionnaire measure being taken immediately before the first treatment of each block and immediately after the second treatment. There were thus a total of 16 measures. The blocks of treatment were presented in a balanced design in order to try to counteract the effects of systematic trends in the illness.

Table 6 shows that the course of the various symptoms differed considerably, especially the phobic and depressive symptoms. The former show very little and the latter a substantial amount of change, ending in recovery.

We have here the basis of our first generalisation; that depressive and phobic anxiety symptoms can fluctuate independently of each other during the course of an affective illness. The results of the three other cases of affective disorder which we have so far published (Shapiro, 1961a and 1963; Shapiro *et al.*, 1962) are consistent with this generalisation. We might, to some degree at least, be dealing with two separate illnesses, each demanding its own separate explanation and treatment.

Our main interest is in the difference between the effects of the two kinds of treatment. Our analysis of variance indicated that differences in the effects of the two treatments did not vary significantly in size from symptom to symptom. We therefore,

TABLE 6

Raw Data (only Phobic and Depressive Symptoms Shown)

		There are four possible scores:					10 is equivalent to illness and 2 to recovery											
								Occasions									Summary of content	
No.		2	3	4	5	6	7	8	9	10	11	12	13	14	15	16	17	$\bar{X}$	
1.		10	10	10	10	10	10	10	10	10	10	10	10	10	10	10	10	10·0	shops-thinking
2.		10	10	10	10	10	10	10	10	10	10	10	10	10	10	10	10	10·0	shops-running out
3.		10	10	10	10	10	10	10	10	10	10	10	7	10	10	10	10	9·9	walks
4.		10	10	7	10	10	10	10	10	10	10	7	10	10	10	10	10	9·6	garden
5.		10	10	10	10	10	10	10	10	10	10	10	10	7	7	7	7	9·2	meeting people
6.		10	10	10	10	10	10	10	10	10	10	7	10	5	10	10	2	9·0	falling fear
	$\bar{x}$	10	10	9·5	10	10	10	10	10	10	10	9·0	9·5	8·7	9·5	9·5	8·2		
20.		10	10	7	5	5	7	5	5	7	5	5	10	5	10	·5	2	6·4	guilt
21.		10	10	7	10	5	7	7	10	5	5	5	5	5	10	2	2	6·4	interest
22.		7	10	5	5	2	5	7	10	7	5	5	5	7	7	7	2	6·0	energy
23.		10	10	2	7	2	2	5	2	7	5	5	5	2	10	5	2	5·1	future
	$\bar{x}$	9·2	10	5·2	6·7	3·5	5·2	6·0	6·7	6·5	5·0	5·0	6·2	4·0	9·2	4·7	2·0		

for the purpose of analysis, thought it permissible to add together the results for all the items. The outcome is reported in Fig. 1. From this graph the following results emerge:

(i) Each form of treatment produced immediate beneficial effects. This was also apparent clinically, the patient often appearing to get better, during a treatment session, before our very eyes.

(ii) the delayed effect of rational training appeared always to be that of relapse, while those of nondirective psychotherapy appeared to be variable, with the average effect being that of further improvement.

We have here, the basis of a second generalisation; that a psychological treatment session sets in motion a process which lasts at least a few days, which can develop in any direction, and which can reverse its direction as time goes on.

Another single case experiment, which was a forerunner of our present programme of research, produced results quite consistent with this generalisation, though the detailed manifestations were quite different; so too were the symptoms and nature of the treatments (Shapiro and Ravenette, 1959).

CONCLUSIONS

We see that a therapeutic experiment on a single case can produce results which are psychologically meaningful, and which present precise problems for further investigation. However, there are many weaknesses in the experiment. For example:

(1) For reasons beyond our control we did not continue with further manipulations of those variables which appeared to be producing definite effects, such as the differences in the immediate and delayed effects of the two kinds of treatment. We have now begun to carry out long term experiments.

(2) We did nothing to ensure the reproducibility and measurability of the treatments.

Two additional facts should be mentioned. The first is that the patient had begun a course of treatment with imipramine one week before the experiment started. The drug might have been

Average scores on the personal questionnaire
on 17 occasions of testing

N = Non-directive
T = Training
I = "Immediate" measures
D = "Delayed" measures

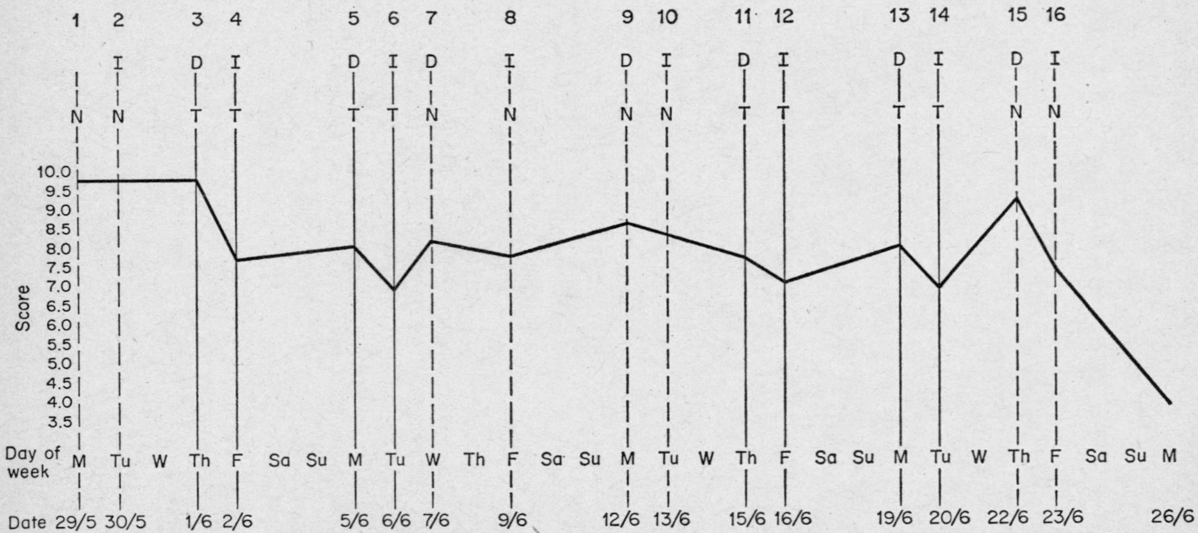

a factor in producing the fluctuations in relation to the independent variable. The second is that the patient continued, nearly two years after the end of the experiment, to show fluctuations of the affective aspects of her illness. The downward trend during the four week experiment could therefore have been part of an overall fluctuation which had little to do with the treatments. However, the essential findings of regular immediate improvements after the application of treatments, and the regular subsequent relapses after behaviour therapy, still remain to be explained and further investigated.

We can best end with a direct quotation from Claude Bernard (p. 14): "In the experimental sciences all progress is measured by improvement in the means of investigation. The whole future of experimental medicine depends on creating a method of research which may be applied fruitfully to the study of vital phenomena whether in a normal or abnormal state."

REFERENCES

BERNARD, C. *An Introduction to the Study of Experimental Medicine.* Reprinted by Dover Publication, New York, 1865.

CHRISTIE, R., HAVEL, J., and SEIDENBERG, B. *J. Abnorm. Soc. Psychol. 56,* 143–159, 1958.

CRONBACH, L. J. *Educ. Psychol. Meas. 10,* 3–31, 1950.

FISKE, D. W. *Educ. Psychol. Meas. 17,* 453, 1957.

GOODENOUGH, F. L. The Measurement of Mental Growth in Childhood, in *Manual of Child Psychology* (Ed. by L. Carmichael), J. J. Wiley, 1946.

JONES, H. G. *J. Abnorm. Soc. Psychol. 52,* 414–419, 1956.

LANDIS, C. and KATZ, S. E. *J. Appl. Psychol. 18,* 343–356, 1934.

SHAPIRO, M. B. *Brit. J. Med. Psychol. 34,* 151–155, 1961a.

SHAPIRO, M. B. *Brit. J. Med. Psychol. 34,* 355–362, 1961b.

SHAPIRO, M. B. The Personal Questionnaire—An Abbreviated Manual. Unpublished, 1961c.

SHAPIRO, M. B. A Clinical Approach to Fundamental Research with Special Reference to the Study of the Single Patient, in *Basic Research Techniques in Psychiatry* (Ed. by P. Sainsbury and N. Kreitman), Oxford University Press, 1963.

SHAPIRO, M. B., NEUFELD, I. and POST, F. *Psychological Reports 10,* 590, 1962.

SHAPIRO, M. B., MARKS, I. M. and FOX, B. *Brit. J. Soc. Clin. Psychol. 2,* 81–93, 1963.

SHAPIRO, M. B. and RAVENETTE, T. *J. Ment. Sci. 105,* 295–312, 1959.

13

A Case Study in a Behavioral Analysis of Psychotherapy*

EDWARD J. MURRAY

Psychotherapy is of considerable interest to many psychologists today. This is partly because psychotherapy is the only rational approach to the treatment of neuroses and psychoses. It is also because psychotherapy is a unique source of data about some of the most important and elusive processes of human behavior. Yet, there is much we need to learn about psychotherapy. It is not clear why only some patients improve. Current research using measures before and after therapy, or comparing therapy with no-therapy, yields little useful information; such an approach establishes no relationship between what actually occurs during therapy and the outcome. Thus, there is no rationale for gradually improving tactics or understanding the changes in various kinds of patients. In spite of the general descriptions of therapy that are available, it is not clear just what happens between a therapist and his patient. To some extent this is due to the complexity and the number of the events in therapy. In addition, we have to contend with the subjectivity of the therapist's report. What is needed is an objective behavioral description of psychotherapy. Such a description must be comprehensive enough to capture the important events and yet simple enough to clarify the complexity of the events. With an adequate description of the events in psychotherapy, studies on the prediction of therapeutic progress from psychological tests, as well as studies on the evaluation of therapy using outside criteria, will take on new meaning and exert more influence on therapeutic conduct. The purpose of this paper is to describe a first step which was taken

* Reprinted from the *Journal of Abnormal and Social Psychology*, 1954, Vol. 49, pp. 305–310, by permission of the author and the publisher.

in the direction of an adequate description of psychotherapy.

Many events occur during psychotherapy. Those which are readily observable may be grouped as physiological, gross behavioral, and verbal. All three groups have been studied (e.g., *3, 10*) and should be studied further. However, verbal behavior seems to be most critical from many points of view. There have been studies on the grammatical and formal properties of verbal behavior in therapy (e.g., *2*), which are interesting in many ways but do not seem to be related to the major theories of personality in any determinate way. The content or meaning functions of verbalization seem much more relevant. The general method for studying such material is called content analysis. The research on psychotherapy done by the Rogers group (*10*) uses content analysis. However, in content analysis the categories which one selects are determined by theory. The theory guiding the Rogerian content analysis appears to be a vague perceptual schema. The content analysis which we are developing is guided by two other points of view: psychoanalytic theory and learning theory. In this context the most relevant categories are those concerned with motivation and defense. Thus, we propose to study the content of verbal behavior in psychotherapy with respect to underlying motives and defenses. This study illustrates this approach with one psychotherapy patient.

A CASE STUDY

The patient was seen for 17 hours in an outpatient clinic. All hours except the thirteenth were phonographically recorded. The first hour was omitted because it consisted of history taking. The patient was referred by the medical clinic. His complaint was that "he has trouble getting to sleep at night—feels that if he falls asleep he may die. He is tremendously threatened but can't say what he is threatened by." At the time of the first interview the patient was described by the therapist as follows:

> The patient is a well built, good looking young man of 24. His family was once well-to-do, he's a college graduate, and he's now working in a real estate firm. . . . His parents were divorced when he was eight after a protracted period of arguments which the pa-

tient remembers as painful to him. Apparently his mother was unfaithful and a good deal of the dispute was about this. The patient also remembers being taunted about his mother's behavior by one of his companions. Before the divorce the entire family moved about and finally lived with the maternal grandmother. He was surrounded by dominating and pampering females. He now relates this to a "complex" of going from person to person for aid. After the divorce he lived with his aunt. His mother remarried, had a child, who is now nine, and moved in with the patient and his aunt, which is the present home situation. His mother was harsh to him and he developed a distaste for her. He wanted to be different from her and rejected her "emotional" kind of living in favor of a "logical and rational approach." He adjusted to school and social relations with boys very easily. He tended, though, to be a teacher's pet in grammar school. He did well in science and math in high school and started out in biology at college. Upon his return to college after the war he changed to the social sciences taking his degree in history. His relations with girls were extremely innocent until he went in the army. He masturbated during adolescence in spite of guilt and fear about it. The army's attitude about masturbation enabled him to overcome a good deal of this guilt. While in the army he went out with a college girl without ever having intercourse, avoiding the kind of girls with whom he might have had sex and avoiding one situation with this girl which might have led to sex. While overseas he did have some sexual relationships. Generally he seems very cooperative and well motivated.

Therapy was mainly supportive but included interpretations about the defensive nature of his physical complaints and the hostility which arose when he became dependent. A permissive attitude toward the expression of hostility was maintained.

After a considerable period of trial and error, two main categories were selected for content analysis: *hostility* and *defense* statements. The hostility category was divided into six subcategories of hostility: (*a*) mother, (*b*) aunt, (*c*) other people, (*d*) general situations and groups, (*e*) the therapist, and (*f*) a vague "at home" (referring to one or more persons in his home). The defense category was composed of: (*a*) intellectual defensive statements which included the patient's views on philosophy, science, current events, etc., and (*b*) complaints about a wide variety of physical symptoms and discomforts. Everything else was considered irrelevant.

The unit scored was called a statement. This was either a simple sentence or the meaning phrases of a more complicated sentence. Each statement was judged as belonging to one of the several categories. The main measure was the number of statements in a given category for each hour. Relationships from hour to hour between categories, and between categories and the behavior of the therapist, were determined.

The record of each hour was played very slowly, and each statement was judged either as belonging to one of the eight categories or as irrelevant. A reliability study with three other judges scoring the same hour showed that the categories were defined in a way which was precise enough for teaching other people the method. The reliability was high when the eight categories were compared ($r = .86$, .89, and .91; $p < .01$ in all cases), and even higher when the irrelevant category was added ($r = .94$, .95, and .98; $p < .01$ in all cases).

HOSTILITY AND DEFENSES

Expressing hostility was a major problem for the patient. In the summary of the treatment, the therapist says, "his problems today seem centered around dependency and concomitant resentment." However, the therapist did feel that some progress was made in his ability to express his hostility as well as to see its relationship with his dependency. If the patient had trouble expressing hostility, then his hostility must have aroused anxiety. From the theory of conflict (*1*, *4*) we would predict that if hostility is inhibited by anxiety, then, if anxiety is reduced by the permissive attitude of the therapist, the overt manifestations of hostility should increase while the overt manifestations of anxiety should decrease. In this study it is assumed that the hostility statements are the overt manifestation of hostility, and the defense statements the overt manifestation of anxiety. Figure 1 shows the hostility and defense statements throughout the course of psychotherapy. It can be seen that hostility increases and defenses decrease. Moreover, the hour-to-hour fluctuations show a true reciprocal relationship which strengthens the conflict analysis. The crisscrossing from Hour 4 to Hour 5 takes place in between the part of the therapy when defenses were high and the later part when the expression of hostility was high. The correlation is negative and highly reliable ($r = -.73$, $p < .01$).

However, the objection might be raised that this is not a dy-

Fig. 1. Frequency of hostility and defense statements throughout therapy.

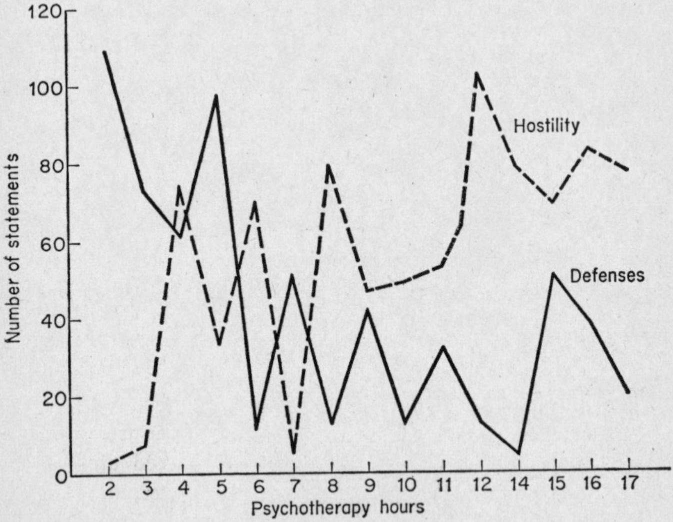

namic relationship between the two categories because the total number of statements is limited and when one category goes up the other must come down. This is not the case, because, with the exception of one hour, pooled hostility and defense statements never constituted more than 60 per cent of the total statements of one hour. An objection which can be made to this is that there may be nothing unique about the hostility-defense relationship if the residual or irrelevant statements also correlate with either hostility or defenses. This objection is ruled out by the fact that the residual is not correlated with hostility ($r = -.20$) or with defenses ($r = .19$). Another objection which might be raised is that, since the total number of statements varied from hour to hour because of differences in the patient's rate of speech, the length of pauses, and the number of therapist's remarks, the relationship is an artifact of the different totals. That this is not the case is shown in Fig. 2, where the percentage of the total number of hostility and defense statements is plotted.[1] In this form, hostility is still negatively and highly

Fig. 2. Percentage of hostility and defense statements throughout therapy.

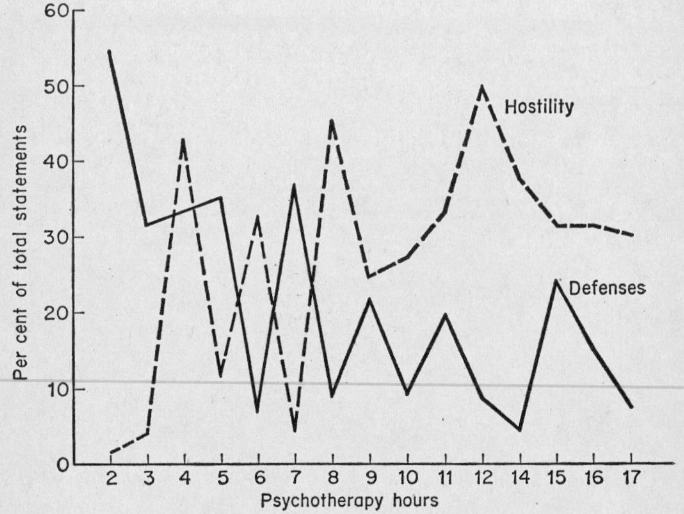

reliably correlated with defenses ($r = -.75$, $p < .01$). Hostility in percentage form correlates very highly with hostility in the frequency form in Fig. 1 ($r = .96$, $p < .01$). This is also true of defenses ($r = .94$, $p < .01$).

We feel that this result strongly suggests that the patient's anxiety about expressing hostility was decreased as a result of the therapist's activity and/or inactivity. However, this may be limited only to the therapeutic situation; outside observations are needed to demonstrate any more general conclusion. The verbal changes shown here may or may not be indicative of fundamental emotional change. Here again, other evidence is needed. It is also conceivable that this hostility was a defense against a

[1] The results presented in Figs. 3, 4, and 5 also show little change when plotted in percentage form.

more anxiety-arousing sexual problem. But in any event, the lawfulness of the change is encouraging for the usefulness of the method.

THE DISPLACEMENT OF HOSTILITY

An examination of the occurrence of statements in the subcategories of hostility from hour to hour reveals a sequence of persons toward whom hostility is directed rather than a global display on each hour. Figure 3 shows hostility to mother, aunt,

Fig. 3. Hostility statements referring to mother, aunt, and others-general throughout therapy.

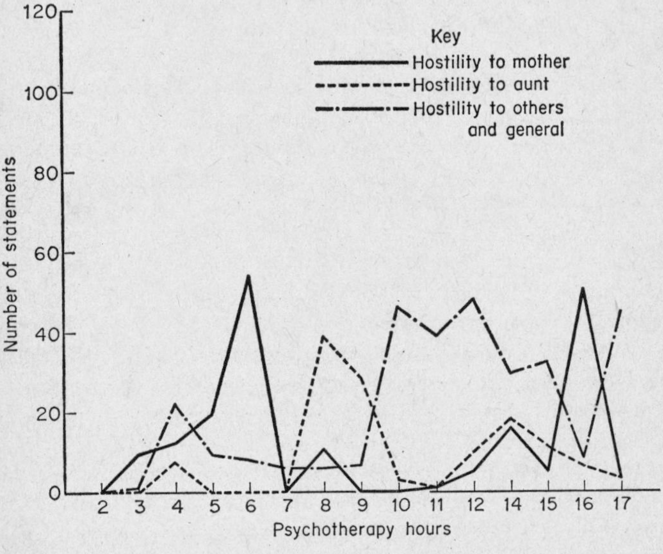

and a combined "others" and "general." The sequence strongly suggests displacement. From a psychoanalytic point of view we would expect the mother to be the recipient of the most basic hostility. Mother, aunt, and others form a meaningful gradient of generalization. The patient's hostility to his mother gradually increased up to Hour 6. The therapist's summary of Hour 6 says, "he revealed that his mother had punished him for masturbating. She also forced food upon him and punished him for not eating promptly. He was 'too little to fight back' but did act in a spiteful way several times. He described other hostilities and retaliations with respect to his mother." The following hour showed little hostility. Then for several hours he expressed hostility to his aunt. This is viewed as primarily a displacement from the mother, although the aunt elicited her own share of hostility. Following this there was a displacement to other people. We expected the sequence to reverse itself, i.e., after the hostility to others, hostility would be expressed first to the aunt again and finally to the mother again. However, a dramatic external event took place between Hours 15 and 16: his aunt was suddenly taken to the hospital for an emergency cancer operation. The therapist says that during Hour 16, "after considerable struggle he finally stated an ambivalency about the event." Furthermore, his hostility to his mother was increased because she had hinted that if the aunt died, *she* would take over the home.

It should be noted that the learning analysis of displacement (*5*), which has been confirmed in several animal experiments (*6, 7, 9*), does not predict sequences of hostility to various objects. Since it is desirable to make such predictions, we embarked on an extension of displacement theory (*8*) and an experimental investigation, in collaboration with Mr. Mitchell Berkun of displacement with animals in a free-choice situation. Suffice it to say that if rats are both rewarded and punished at a given goal so as to establish a conflict, they will still approach that goal part way before displacing to another goal. This is an example of how precise data from psychotherapy can influence theories of behavior based on animal work.

The fact that hostility was directed toward people who were further and further displaced provides an alternative explanation for the general increase in hostility throughout therapy. If expressing hostility to these people aroused less anxiety than expressing hostility to his mother, we would expect more and more hostility as therapy progressed. Probably *both* displacement and a general reduction of anxiety because of the treatment operated to permit hostility to increase. The hostility expressed to the patient's mother in Hour 16 was much stronger and was concerned with much more recent events than was the hostility in

Hour 6. Thus, there was a therapeutic effect. Indeed, expressing hostility to relatively unimportant people may be therapeutically valuable because it is less fearful. In learning theory terms, fear is extinguished in the displaced situation and these extinction effects are generalized back to the fear in the primary conflict situation. In the experiment mentioned above, the rats returned to the original goal after making unpunished goal responses in the displaced situation.

DEFENSES

The two defense categories seemed to operate as alternate members of a defensive armamentarium. In Fig. 4 it can be

Fig. 4. The interaction of intellectual and physical complaint defenses and the effects of interpretations during the first portion of therapy.

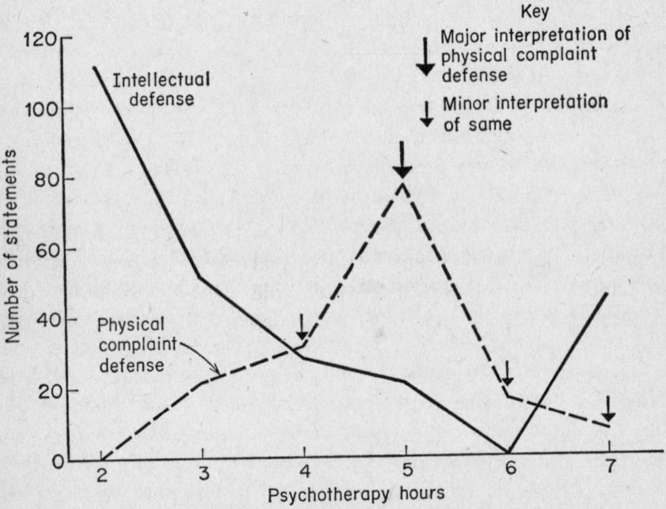

seen that the intellectual defense was high at the outset and decreased throughout the first part of therapy. This intellectual defense was never interpreted. The physical complaint defense increased as the intellectual defense decreased. After the major interpretation in Hour 5, the physical complaint defense dropped off sharply. In Hour 6 both defenses were low, and this hour proved to be especially fruitful as was noted above. This expression of hostility also increased his anxiety, and the following hour was a dull one. Moreover, with the physical complaint defense interpreted the noninterpreted intellectual defense increased in a compensatory way in this subsequent hour. Both defenses decreased during the rest of psychotherapy and show no distinguishing features as far as the number of responses is concerned. The interpretation of the physical complaints may have functioned as a punishment, or may have established insight. Further indices are needed to distinguish between the two possibilities.

There is also a possibility that the two defenses had different functions. The intellectual defense was more assertive and self-aggrandizing. It may have been a way of telling the therapist that he was masculine or mature. On the other hand, the physical complaints had a pleading and ingratiating tone. This defense may have been motivated by feminine or dependent needs. However, both may be viewed as motivated by anxiety and both served the function of avoiding talk about conflict areas.

Fortunately, we examined another case which showed some striking similarities to this one. The general personality picture was the same as the present case. In addition, the two chief defenses were similar to the physical complaints and intellectualizations characterizing our present case. The second patient had physical complaints, although he had more insight into their psychogenesis. A category comprising physical complaints and more psychologically phrased feelings of tension, conflict, and blocking was defined. The intellectual defense was quite similar to the first case. Figure 5 shows the course of physical, etc. defensive statements and intellectual defensive statements throughout the eight hours of therapy. This second patient began with physical complaints which decreased from Hour 1 to Hour 3 without interpretation. As the physical complaints decreased, the intellectual defense increased. This was interpreted in a punitive way in Hour 2 and, less severely, in Hours 3 and 4. Both defenses were low in Hours 3 and 4 and it was in these hours, both in our opinion and in the unsolicited opinion of the therapist, that the most important hostile material came out. In Hour 5 it was

Fig. 5. The interaction of intellectual and physical complaint defenses and the effects of interpretations throughout the therapy of a second patient.

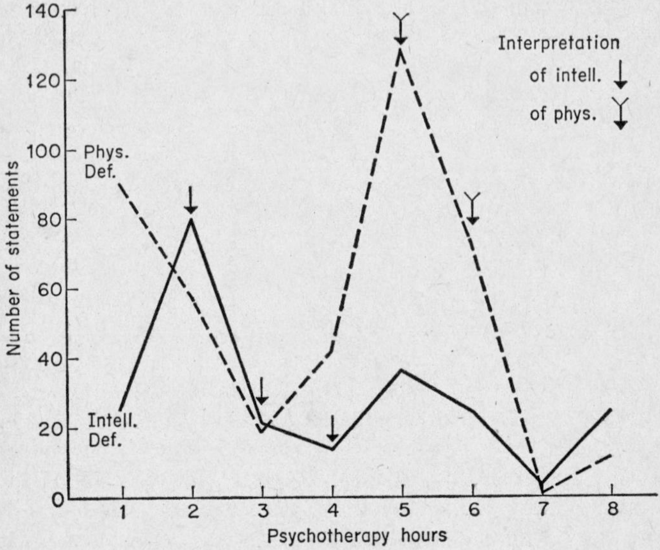

the uninterpreted defense—physical complaints—that showed the greatest increase. In this case, the therapist then proceeded to interpret the physical complaint defense on Hours 5 and 6. Both defenses were low for the last two hours.

This second case in a sense provides a natural experimental control for the first case. In the first case intellectual defenses were highest at first and decreased without interpretation; in the second case this was true of physical complaints. In the first case physical complaints supplanted intellectual defenses; in the second case intellectual defenses supplanted physical complaints. In the first case the physical complaints met with the disapproval of the therapist; in the second case this was true of intellectualizations. In both cases the punitively interpreted defenses decreased. In both cases important hostile material emerged when both physical complaints and intellectualizations were low. In both cases the expression of hostility was followed by an upswing in the uninterpreted defense. These results strengthen our belief that the physical complaints and intellectualizations are alternate defenses against anxiety. They also tend to confirm the general conflict analysis we have made. The increase in defenses after the expression of hostility may be related to the "negative therapeutic effect" (*1*). We may also tentatively formulate the hypothesis that, with this kind of patient, uninterpreted (or unpunished) defenses have a greater probability of occurrence when anxiety is increased than interpreted (or punished) defenses. It is obvious that much more evidence is needed before making any definite conclusions.

SUMMARY AND CONCLUSIONS

In our present state of knowledge about psychotherapy, final conclusions should be avoided. Therefore, it is with trepidation that we approach the task of making a comprehensive summary statement about our illustrative case. This is true even though the therapy was brief and the changes were probably not fundamental. We might ask about the success of this case. The therapist does not sound optimistic in his summary: "The patient now has insight into his problems but can't extricate himself from them. Because of a general character weakness it is improbable that short term therapy will be of much more value." But our feeling is that it is important to understand what has happened during these interviews, whether or not the therapy was eminently successful. We feel that our objective description aids in this. Here is a tentative recapitulation of the case in terms of the data presented in this study.

The patient began treatment with a good deal of anxiety and subsequent defensiveness. His defensiveness decreased as a result of a combination of permissiveness about hostility and punitiveness about defenses on the part of the therapist. As this occurred he expressed strong hostility to his mother. This expression of hostility led to an increase in anxiety and defensivenes. The defense which increased was the one not previously punished by the therapist. Subsequently, hostility was displaced further and further away from his mother. Hostility to displaced objects was stronger because it aroused less anxiety. It is possible that because of the unpunished expression of hostility to the displaced objects, the patient was able later in therapy, when environmental factors precipitated it, to express hostility about his mother much more strongly, at least in the therapeutic situation.

Although this integration involves several assumptions, we feel it is strongly supported by the data. It will be noted that the statements made in the summary concern motivational and defensive shifts. This is what the categories were set up to measure. Other events, such as the establishment of insight, require other kinds of categories. Thus, we offer no evidence to support the therapist's opinion that the patient understood the relationship between his hostility and his dependency at the end of therapy.

This preliminary study has been presented to illustrate the kinds of results which can be obtained by studying psychotherapy carefully and quantitatively. We feel that it also demonstrates the applicability of principles derived from animal and human experimentation to complex human behavior. On the other hand, it is only data as clear as these that will stimulate experimental work and modify existing theories. We also hope that this study has indicated some of the difficulties involved in a behavioral analysis of psychotherapy. Cases do not miraculously become comparable when studied quantitatively. New cases are expected to present as many problems as they solve. Nor do we feel that all of the important events in psychotherapy can be described by this method. Indeed, many important things in this case have been ignored. But, as this methed becomes more refined and as equally objective measures are added to it, we feel that our understanding of psychotherapy, and human behavior in general, will be furthered.

REFERENCES

1. Dollard, J., & Miller, N. E. *Personality and psychotherapy.* New York: McGraw-Hill, 1950.
2. Grummon, D. L. An investigation into the use of grammatical and psycho-grammatical categories of language for the study of personality and psychotherapy. Unpublished Ph.D. dissertation, Univer. of Chicago, 1950.
3. Lasswell, H. D. Certain prognostic changes during trial (psychoanalytic) interviews. *Psychoanal. Rev.,* 1936, *23,* 241–247.
4. Miller, N. E. Experimental studies of conflict. In J. McV. Hunt

(Ed.), *Personality and the behavior disorders.* New York: Ronald, 1944. Pp. 431–465.

5. MILLER, N. E. Theory and experiment relating psychoanalytic displacement to stimulus response generalization. *J. abnorm. soc. Psych.,* 1948, *43,* 155–178.
6. MILLER, N. E., & KRAELING, DORIS. Displacement: greater generalization of approach than avoidance in a generalized approach-avoidance conflict. *J. exp. Psychol.,* 1952, *43,* 217–221.
7. MILLER, N. E., & MURRAY, E. J. Displacement and conflict: learnable drive as a basis for the steeper gradient of avoidance than of approach. *J. exp. Psychol.,* 1952, *43,* 227–231.
8. MURRAY, E. J. Displacement in psychotherapy. Paper read at East. Psychol. Ass., Boston, 1955.
9. MURRAY, E. J. & MILLER, N. E. Displacement: steeper gradient of generalization of avoidance than of approach with age of habit controlled. *J. exp. Psychol.,* 1952, *43,* 222–226.
10. ROGERS, C. R. *Client-centered therapy.* Boston: Houghton Mifflin, 1951.

14

Aversive Control of Self-Injurious Behavior in a Psychotic Boy*

B. G. TATE and GEORGE S. BAROFF

Summary—Two studies are reported which indicate how quickly and effectively chronic self-injurious behavior was controlled in a 9-yr-old blind psychotic boy. In the first study, the self-injurious responses were punished by contingent withdrawal of human physical contact. In the second study, response-contingent electric shock was employed.

INTRODUCTION

There have been many attempts to explain self-injurious behavior (Cain, 1961; Dollard *et al.,* 1939; Freud, 1954; Goldfarb, 1945; Greenacre, 1954; Hartmann *et al.,* 1949; Sandler, 1964). It has been labeled masochism, auto-aggression, self-aggression, and self-destructive behavior. The present authors prefer the term self-injurious behavior because it is more descriptive and less interpretive. Self-injurious behavior (SIB) does not imply an attempt to destroy, nor does it suggest aggression; it simply means behavior which produces physical injury to the individual's own body. Typically SIB is composed of a series of self-injurious responses (SIRs) that are repetitive and sometimes rhythmical, often with no obvious reinforcers, and therefore similar to stereotyped behavior. Common types of SIB are forceful head-banging, face slapping, punching the face and head, and scratching and biting one's body.

A patient who emits SIRs at high frequency and/or magnitude is particularly difficult to work with because the behavior inter-

* Reprinted from *Behavior Research and Therapy,* 1966, Vol. 4, pp. 281–287, by permission of the authors and the publisher.

feres with the production of more desirable responses and there is always the risk of severe and permanent physical injury, e.g. head and eye damage. Usually such patients must be physically restrained or maintained on heavy dosages of drugs. Lovaas *et al.* (1964), however, successfully employed punishment in the form of painful electric shock to dramatically reduce the frequency of SIRs in several schizophrenic children. Ball (1965) used the same technique with a severely retarded girl and achieved similar results.

The present paper describes two punishment procedures used to control SIB in a psychotic boy. In Study I, punishment was withdrawal of human physical contact contingent on a SIR. In Study II, punishment was response-contingent painful electric shock. Following a description of the subject, the procedures and results of Studies I and II are presented, followed by a report on related behavioral changes and a general discussion.

SUBJECT

Sam was a 9-yr-old, blind male who was transferred for evaluation and treatment on a research basis from an out-of-state psychiatric hospital to Murdoch Center, a state institution for the mentally retarded. At the age of 5 he was diagnosed as autistic and was hospitalized. For the next 4 yr he received group and individual psychotherapy, and drug therapy with no long-term benefit. Drugs were used in an effort to control self-injurious behavior, screaming, and hyperactivity.

The SIB began at about the age of 4 and consisted of face slapping. By age 9, his SIB repertoire included banging his head forcefully against floors, walls, and other hard objects, slapping his face with his hands, punching his face and head with his fists, hitting his shoulder with his chin, and kicking himself. Infrequently he would also pinch, bite, and scratch others.

At age 8, bilateral cataracts, a complete detachment of the left retina, and partial detachment of the right retina were discovered. An ophthalmologist has suggested that the cataracts were probably congenital but were not noticed until they matured and that the retinal detachments were likely caused by head-banging. The cataract in the right eye was removed soon after its discovery, leaving Sam with some light-dark vision and possibly some movement perception.

Upon arrival at Murdoch Center, Sam was assigned a room in the infirmary and drugs were immediately discontinued. Casual observations were made for the first 2 weeks while he was adapting to his new environment. Following the adaptation period, eighteen 30-min daily observation periods were conducted during which a female research assistant held Sam, tried to interest him in games, and ignored all SIRs. These observations yielded a median daily average SIR rate of 2.3/min (range: 0.9–7.9/min). A second type of observation consisted of 5-min periods four times a day at random intervals. Over a 26-day period the median daily average SIR rate was 1.7/min (range: 0.3–4.1/min). SIB, therefore, was a frequent form of behavior observed under a wide variety of situations.

Observations also revealed the following: Sam had a firm hematoma approximately 7 cm in diameter on his forehead—a result of previous head-banging. His speech was limited to jargon and to approximately twenty words usually spoken in a high-pitched, whining manner and often inappropriately used. He was not considered autistic at this time because he obviously enjoyed and sought bodily contact with others. He would cling to people and try to wrap their arms around him, climb into their laps and mold himself to their contours. When left alone and free, he would cry, scream, flail his arms about, and hit himself or bang his head. When fully restrained in bed he was usually calm, but often engaged in head-rolling and hitting his chin against his shoulder.

STUDY I: CONTROL BY WITHDRAWAL AND REINSTATEMENT OF HUMAN PHYSICAL CONTACT

Early observations of Sam strongly indicated that physical contact with people was reinforcing to him and that being alone, particularly when he was standing or walking, was aversive. Study I was undertaken in an effort to learn if a procedure of withdrawing physical contact when a SIR occurred and reinstating the contact after a brief interval during which no SIRs occurred could be used to control Sam's SIB.

Procedure

Study I began on the fourth day following the end of the 26-day observation period mentioned. During the 3 weeks preceding the commencement of the study Sam was restrained in his bed except for morning baths given by attendants and for daily walks around the campus and through the infirmary corridors with two female research assistants (Es). During the walks Es held Sam's hands and chatted to him and to each other and ignored SIRs.

Study I consisted of twenty daily 20-min sessions run at the same time each day by the same Es. There were five control sessions (SIRs were ignored), followed by five experimental sessions (SIRs were punished), five control sessions, and five experimental sessions.

Control sessions consisted of a walk around the campus with the two Es who chatted with Sam and with each other. Sam walked between them, holding onto a hand of each. When he emitted SIRs the Es ignored them.

Experimental sessions were identical to the control sessions expect that when Sam hit himself, Es jerked their hands free so that he had no physical contact with them. The time-out from physical contact lasted 3 sec following the last SIR. At the end of 3 sec, Es allowed him to grasp their hands and the walk resumed. No comments were made to Sam when a hit occurred —the only responses to the SIR were withdrawal of contact and cessation of talk if Es were talking at the time.

All sessions began when Sam left his room and entered the corridor leading outside the building. The same route around the campus was followed each day. Each session ended while he was outside the building, but the procedure for the particular session was continued until Sam was returned to his room, undressed, placed in bed, and restrained—usually about 12 additional min. Records were kept by one E who silently marked the SIRs on a piece of paper during the walks.

Results of Study I

Virtually all of the SIRs made during the sessions were chin-to-shoulder hits. On a few occasions Sam would punch his head with his fist during punishment but he rarely withdrew his hand from an assistant and hit himself.

Figure 1 presents the average SIRs per min for each day of the study. The median average rate of SIRs for the first 5

Fig. 1. Effect of the punishment procedure of Study I on the daily average frequency of SIRs. On experimental days SIRs were followed by withdrawal of human physical contact and reinstatement of contact after a minimum interval of 3 sec. On control days the SIRs were ignored.

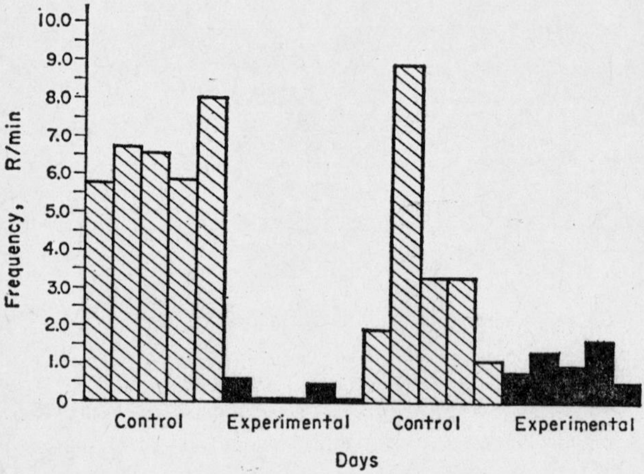

control days was 6.6 responses per min and sharply declined to a median average of 0.1 responses per min for the following 5 experimental days. The response rate recovered somewhat (median average = 3.3) during the second 5 control days and decreased again during the second 5 experimental days (median average = 1.0). The unusually high rate of SIRs on the second day of the second control run was associated with a temper tantrum which lasted about 15 min.

On the experimental days an interesting change in Sam's behavior occurred which was noticed by both Es and the authors.

On control days Sam typically whined, cried, hesitated often in his walk, and seemed unresponsive to the environment in general. His behavior on experimental days was completely different—he appeared to attend more to environmental stimuli, including the Es; there was no crying or whining, and he often smiled. A brief discussion of this change in behavior appears at the end of the paper.

The results of this study indicate that the relatively simple procedure of controlling the contingencies of this chronic SIB produced a dramatic reduction in its frequency. Of interest also are the relative effects of punishing the SIR and ignoring it. These results do not, of course, mean that long-term effects would be the same.

STUDY II: CONTROL BY ELECTRIC SHOCK

Although the SIB could be reduced by response-contingent withdrawal of physical contact, it was decided that the risk of completely destroying the right retina by further head-banging was great enough to preclude the long term use of this method. Parental permission was then obtained for the use of painful electric shock.

The shock apparatus was a stock prod (Sears & Roebuck Number 325971) similar to the one used by Lovaas *et al.* (1964). The prod was a cylinder 58 cm long and 3 cm in diameter containing seven D cells and an induction coil. With fresh batteries approximately 130 v were available at the two 0.48 cm diameter terminals, 1.24 cm apart, projecting from one end of the prod. Shock was administered by turning the induction coil on and touching the terminals to the bare skin of the patient.

Study II began 46 hr after the termination of Study I.

Procedure

For 24 min prior to the administration of electric shock, Sam was allowed a free-responding period. The authors, accompanied by a physician, entered Sam's room, talked to him pleasantly and freed his hands, leaving him lying in bed with both feet restrained. They remained close to his bed while an assistant in an adjoining room recorded each SIR. After 24 min of observing and recording the free-responding behavior, it was explained to Sam that if he continued to hit himself he would be shocked, and the shock would hurt. A shock of approximately 0.5 second duration then immediately followed each SIR. No more comments were made to Sam concerning the shock which was delivered to the lower right leg.

The contingent shock period was continued for 90 min. After the first two shocks were administered, Sam's feet were untied and he was placed in a sitting position in bed. The authors talked pleasantly to him and encouraged him to play with toys. Approximately 1 hr after the first shock he was placed in a rocking chair for 30 min. Sam was then returned to his bed and left alone unrestrained, while being observed for another 90 min over closed-circuit television. Contingent shock was continued, but there was a delay of 30–35 sec between the SIR and the administration of punishment (time required to reach Sam's room from the observation room).

Shock was continued on subsequent days and was sometimes delivered immediately and sometimes delayed 30 sec depending on whether the therapist was with Sam or observing him on television. At night he was restrained in bed at the wrists and ankles with cloth restraints.

Results of Study II

As soon as Sam's hands were released for the 24-min free-responding period he began hitting his face with his fists. The intensity of the SIRs immediately increased as a temper tantrum developed during which he screamed, flailed his arms about wildly, twisted his body about, hit his face and head with his fists, hit his shoulder with his chin, and banged his head with great force against the iron side rail of the bed. The head-banging was so forceful that it was necessary to cushion the blows by placing the authors' hands over the bed rail. The average rate of SIRs during the 6-min temper tantrum was 14.0 per min. During the next 18 min he became calmer and the average rate dropped to 2.0 responses per min.

During the first 90-min contingent shock period a total of

only five SIRs were emitted (average rate = 0.06 responses per min). The shocks produced a startle reaction in Sam and avoidance movements, but no cries. The authors talked to him, praised virtually all non-injurious responses, and generally behaved pleasantly. When led from the bed to the rocking chair, he immediately began crying and flailing his arms. A SIR was promptly followed by a shock and he became calm. A few seconds later he was sitting in the chair and smiling with apparent pleasure. At the end of the 90-min period Sam was returned to his bed and left in it free while being observed over closed-circuit television. Throughout the second 90-min observation period he remained quietly in bed posturing with his hands. Four SIRs were emitted and were followed by delayed shocks. The SIR rate had decreased from 2.0/min in the last minutes of the free responding period to 0.04/min. At the end of the period a meal was offered which he refused. He was then restrained for the night.

The following day Sam was free from 9:00 A.M. until 2:30 P.M. All of this time was spent in bed with toys except for 1 hr in the afternoon during which the authors encouraged him to rock in a rocking chair and walk around his room. Twenty SIRs of light intensity occurred during the 5½-hr period (average rate = 0.06 responses per min). Four of these were followed by immediate shock and the other sixteen by delayed shock.

On the second day following the commencement of shock Sam was free from 8:00 A.M. until 4:30 P.M. There were only fifteen SIRs during the entire day (average rate = 0.03/min) but most of these occurred during one brief period of agitation at noon. He was out of bed about 3 hr being rocked, walked, and entertained with toys.

In the ensuing days Sam's daily activities were gradually increased until he remained out of bed 9 hr a day. He was still restrained at night because of limited personnel available to check him. He began attending physical therapy classes for the severely retarded 3 hr a day where he was encouraged to play with a variety of toys. He now apparently enjoys walks, playground equipment, and playing "games" involving following directions and making discriminations, for example, various objects (ball, book, music box, etc.) are put on a table across the room and he is asked to bring a specific one to E. He is more spontaneous in his activities than he was when he arrived and he is now capable of walking and running alone without clinging to people.

Punishment of SIRs with shock was continued and the decline in rate progressed. Since the beginning of shock 167 days have elapsed. The last observed SIR was emitted on day 147.

OTHER CHANGES IN BEHAVIOR

Sam's intake of food and liquids had undergone an overall decrease since his admission although there were wide day-to-day fluctuations. Three months after his admission (5 days before the use of shock), his weight had decreased by 14 lb (20 per cent). On days when he ate nothing he usually held great quantities of saliva in his mouth for hours—emptying his mouth only by accident or when forced to. In the 36 hr preceding the commencement of shock, Sam ate only a small portion of one meal and drank only 400 ml of liquids. Supper was refused on the day shock was first administered. The following day he drank a small quantity of milk and ate some cereal for breakfast, but all other liquids and food were refused during the day—he had started saving saliva again. In addition he was posturing with his hands most of the day (posturing had been observed before any treatment began).

On the second day following the commencement of shock he refused all food during the morning. At 2:00 P.M., he was again offered juice which he refused. He was then told firmly to drink but he would not open his mouth. It was then discovered that a firm command followed by the buzz of the stock prod (but no shock delivered), would cause him to open his mouth and take the juice, but he then held it in his mouth without swallowing. Again, a command and a buzz produced swallowing. The sequence of "Drink," and "Swallow," was repeated until he had consumed all of the juice. Verbal praise and affectionate pats were used to reinforce each desirable response. With this procedure, command-buzz-reinforcement, he also drank a glass of milk and ate some ice cream. This was the most food he had consumed in 4 days. Only one shock was actually administered—buzzing of the prod was sufficient the other times. This procedure was continued for the evening meal and the following day. On the third day he began eating spontaneously and has continued, although there are still occasions when he has to be prompted. In the following 15 days he gained 10 lb and his weight continues to increase, but at a normal rate.

The posturing was stopped in similar fashion. When, for example, Sam held his hands up instead of down by his sides, he was told firmly to put his hands down, and if he did not, the buzzing of the prod was presented. The act of holding saliva in his mouth was stopped by telling him firmly to swallow and sounding the prod if he did not obey. The same procedure was effective in reducing his clinging to people.

DISCUSSION

Both punishment procedures effectively reduced SIB in this psychotic boy. Aversive control by withdrawal of physical contact was immediately effective both times it was used.

Aversive control by painful electric shock also reduced the SIB immediately and has remained effective over a 6-month period. In addition, it was found that eating behavior could be reinstated, posturing could be stopped, and saliva-saving and clinging could be terminated by firm commands followed by the sound of the shock apparatus if there was no compliance, and followed by social reinforcement if compliance occurred. Over the 6-month period since the inception of shock, its use has decreased. Part of the beneficial effects of punishment by shock obviously were derived from the more stimulating environment provided him following the initial treatment—an environment which could not have been provided had the SIR rate not been suppressed to avoid injury. A secondary gain was probably derived from the marked positive change in behavior of attendants and nurses toward Sam. It should also be noted that punishment by electric shock prevented accidental reinforcement of SIRs. Before any treatment began it was sometimes necessary to interfere with SIRs by holding Sam's arms, a procedure which may have been reinforcing to him. No deleterious effects of the shock were observed.

An intriguing area of speculation is how to account for the complete change in behavior observed on experimental days of Study I and observed often after shock was delivered in Study II. One plausible explanation for the difference in behavior is that the whining, crying, and SIB belong to the same response class and the suppression of SIB also suppresses these other behaviors. Once the undesirable behaviors are suppressed the more desirable ones, e.g. smiling, listening, attending to the environment, and cooperating with others can occur.

Another conjecture is that both types of punishment produce a general arousal in the central nervous system which results in increased attention (Hebb, 1955). Attention to the external environment could account for the cooperative behavior, smiling and apparent listening. This idea is further supported by the immediacy of the punishment effect—not only did SIB, whining, crying, and negativistic behavior cease abruptly, but within seconds the more desirable behaviors emerged.

REFERENCES

BALL, T. S. (1965) Personal communication.

CAIN, A. C. (1961) The presuperego turning inward of aggression. *Psychoanal. Q. 30,* 171–208.

DOLLARD, J., DOOB L. W., MILLER, N. E., MOWRER, O. H. and SEARS, R. R. (1939) *Frustration and Aggression.* Yale University Press, New Haven.

FREUD, A. (1954) Problems of infantile neurosis: a discussion. In *The Psychoanalytic Study of the Child,* Vol. IX. International Universities Press, New York.

GOLDFARB, W. (1945) Psychological privation in infancy. *Am. J. Orthopsychiat. 15,* 247–255.

GREENACRE, P. (1954) Problems of infantile neurosis: a discussion. In *The Psychoanalytic Study of the Child,* Vol. IX. International Universities Press, New York.

HARTMANN, H., KRIS, E. and LOEWENSTEIN, R. M. (1949) Notes on the theory of aggression. In *The Psychoanalytic Study of the Child.* Vols. III–IV. International Universities Press, New York.

HEBB, D. O. (1955) Drives and the C.N.S. (conceptual nervous system). *Psychol. Rev. 62,* 243–254.

LOVAAS, O. I., FREITAG, G., KINDER, M. I., RUBENSTEIN, D. B., SCHAEFFER, B. and SIMMONS, J. B. (1964) *Experimental Studies in*

Childhood Schizophrenia. Developing Social Behavior Using Electric Shock. Paper read at American Psychological Association Annual Convention, Los Angeles, California.

SANDLER, J. (1964) Masochism: an empirical analysis. *Psychol. Bull. 62,* 197–204.

15

An Approach to the Evaluation of Drug Effect During Psychotherapy: A Double-Blind Study of a Single Case*

LEOPOLD BELLAK and J. B. CHASSAN

INTRODUCTION

It is a well known paradox that convincing experiences of clinicians are derived from intensive clinical work with individual patients, while research data are usually obtained from extensive statistical studies of rather large populations of patients and are often rather superficial.

The evaluation of psychotropic drugs shares many problems with the evaluation of psychotherapy: the problem of valid and reliable judgments, the effect of time and the problem of understanding and demonstrating the process of the therapeutic effect, rather than a mere evaluation of the result (*2*). Not the least among these difficulties derive from the procedure of testing various hypotheses by comparing groups of patients in terms of the relative efficacy of two or more medications. The inability to specify particular patient parameters in relation to the statistical results of such studies, the unknown characteristics of the population of patients from which the research subjects are presumably considered as a random sample and the consequent poverty of operational implications of the results of such studies, are among the many difficulties one encounters in what has been called the extensive model of clinical research design.

---

* Reprinted by permission from: Bellak, Leopold and Chassan, J. B., "An approach to the evaluation of drug effect during psychotherapy: a double-blind study of a single case," *Journal of Nervous and Mental Disease,* 139: 20–30.

From another point of view the use of the extensive model has the effect of exaggerating some of the differences in orientation between clinical research and clinical practice with a consequent feeling of alienation from research on the part of many clinicians who might otherwise be strongly motivated towards it. Research in which statistical comparisons are limited to tests between groups of patients ignore what is happening to the individual patient; to the ebb and flow of his symptoms, to their interpretation within a dynamic framework so important to an understanding of individual psychopathology; and to a more definitive understanding of differential drug effects. There has long been abroad in the land of clinical research the notion that comparisons between groups of patients is the *sine qua non* of statistically valid scientific clinical research, and that the study of the individual case must be relegated at best to a status of intuition and the clinical hunch, not capable of statistical testing and validation. For reasons that have been discussed in some detail (*5*, *6*) this view is seen to lack validity in its own right. It has unfortunately tended to perpetuate a basically superficial methodology as a unique prototype for science in clinical research with mental patients.

What we are stating here is not that the extensive model itself is necessarily unscientific nor that when properly and appropriately performed cannot be viewed as a statistically valid approach to clinical investigation; but rather that it is quite limiting, and that the clinical-statistical study of the individual case (*i.e.*, the intensive design) is, at the very least, a much-needed complementary approach. One of us has made a previous attempt to bridge the difficulties between the clinical and the experimental statistically useful approach by the method of repeated short-range predictions and judgments by independent observers after interaction in psychoanalytic interviews (*3*). This study involved not only one psychoanalyst as a clinician but three psychoanalysts working as predictors and three as judges in a complex experimental setting. The controlled sequence of multidimensional observations was thus made in the framework of testing various hypotheses relevant to the population implicitly defined by the parameters of the single case under study.

The purpose of the present report is to demonstrate a method (and its feasibility) for the evaluation of drug efficacy within the context of the single case and particularly within a framework of the process and practice of psychotherapy by one therapist. A recognition of the possible advantages of the use of drugs as an adjunct to analytically-oriented psychotherapy antedates the present age of ataractics, although very little, if any, formal research using the double-blind technique seems to have been done in this area.

Although this study is based on data from only one case, it is not intended to convey the impression that intensive research designs should necessarily be limited to a single case. The essential property of the intensive design is that each patient in a study is observed periodically over some time-span, and that statistical inferences including tests of hypotheses concerning treatment effects are made basically, *within* the data of each case separately, so that if there were, say, six patients in a study, it would be as though one were gathering and analyzing the data from six separate studies. An incidental advantage of having several patients in an intensive design, apart from the larger number of within-patient hypotheses one can then test, is that one can, upon failing to obtain within-patient significance, and depending upon the overall design of the experiment, pool the data in a manner which may still yield a valid statistically significant result, although the particular hypothesis tested in this way will then approach the type of hypothesis tested in an extensive design.

LIMITATIONS

This investigation was set up mainly as a short, preliminary study to determine whether some of the procedures (as those described below) necessary to establish a tight double-blind study for the evaluation of the efficacy of a drug such as chlordiazepoxide (Librium) by the use of an intensive design, and during a segment of psychotherapy, are feasible. Since this was the primary goal rather than that of testing hypotheses concerning the efficacy of the medication by this method at this time, no attempt was made to provide an adequate time-span for the patient under study to provide a reasonable probability of obtaining statistically significant effects. For the purpose of determining feasibility it was thus estimated that a sequence of ten weekly interviews would be adequate. Contrary to expectations, we did obtain at least borderline significance in a number of the eight variables which were observed at each interview, favoring the active medication over the proverbial identical-appearing placebo, and in each of the remaining variables the averages on chlordiazepoxide showed less psychopathology than the corresponding averages on placebo.

Despite these particular results, however, the short time-span, and concomitantly, the small number of observations such as were made in this study would in general have to be regarded as a serious limitation on the chance of securing sufficient data to obtain statistically significant differences toward the detection of true effects. This is, of course, a widely recognized limitation of a very small sample, whether the sample size is based on the number of patients in an extensive design, or on the number of observations along the time-axis of the individual case in the intensive design.

There is also a second danger, usually not explicitly stated, and perhaps not generally recognized, but nevertheless implicit in the use of very small samples. This can arise even when an apparently statistically significant result *does* occur, in both the intensive design when a too-small time-sample of the single-case is taken and in the extensive design when too few patients are used. This second difficulty arises from the influence that one or two extremely biased observations, say, can have on a total, or on an average, based on a very small number of observations. The term, biased observations, in this context would apply as well to instances of cases that really do not belong in a study, or to the effect of extremely atypical events (as can be the case in a single-case study based on a small time-sample) as well as to isolated instances of observer bias in both types of designs. In larger samples the influence of the singular atypical observation will obviously be less important.

ASPECTS OF THE DESIGN

Selection of Patient Variables and Description of the Patient

One of the advantages of intensive design is that, in focusing on the individual case, it encourages the use of items for rating and evaluating psychopathology which, at least in the view of the clinician who is treating and observing the patient, are specific *to* the patient. This is in contrast to the approach which is so often used in the extensive design when patients with diverse symptomatology and dynamic patterns are thrust, as it were, onto a single hyper-dimensionalized rating sheet and in which statistical analyses take no account of highly relevant individual differences in the interpretability of the direction of a patient's movement along one or another particular scale item, or dimension.

The patient selected for this study was known to the senior author through a previous course of treatment. The patient suffered from acute anxiety, feelings of depersonalization and marked dissociation. From this previous contact, years before this study, together with observations made during an interview with her a week before the beginning of the study proper, he constructed a set of eight variables as follows:

1) Evidence of primary process (thought disorder)
2) Anxiety
3) Confusion
4) Depression
5) Hostility
6) "Sexual flooding"
7) Depersonalization
8) Ability to communicate usefully

Each of these items was rated by the senior author at the end of each session of psychotherapy on a six-point scale. For each of the first seven items a zero rating indicated a complete absence of pathology and a rating of five represented the most severe level of pathology. For item 8, a zero represented the most pathological state, and a five the most favorable.

The rating scale used in this case was subjective in the following sense. The individual patient had already been well known to the therapist from a previous course of treatment and was used as her own frame of reference. The previous experience with this patient was one of the reasons for using her in the present study. Previous work with scales involving approximately the same variables, under controlled circumstances (*2, 4*) had given the therapist a measure of confidence about judgment reliability. Definitions used in this previous work constituted the conceptual point of reference. Nevertheless, in the absence of independent observers this procedure remains crude and strictly an exploratory approach. There is no reason, however, why the same procedure using independent ratings of taped interview material cannot easily be made methodologically acceptable.

A few brief concrete examples may be useful. With regard to depersonalization, lack of any reported experiences of this nature (by this highly intelligent patient who has had experience with such feelings as well as an excellent verbal facility for describing them) was considered a reasonable basis for scoring depersonalization zero. A rating of five was given when the patient's report included such material as the following:

> I feel odd. I feel strange, as if I were drunk, in a daze. I took a walk and everything looked unreal and I began to feel quite sick. . . . I had very odd thoughts and the perspective of the ground was very strange. I felt, I am not sure whether I am there. I look in the mirror. I have the feeling of a stuffed head. Lights bother me, outdoors looks very strange. I feel as if I were someone else.

Intermediate ratings of depersonalization were made when the patient mentioned only some of these complaints; the ratings were based on the frequency of these phenomena since the previous interview and the degree of disturbance they caused. They were sometimes crippling, and at other times transitory and only mildly interfering.

With regard to the primary process ratings, contamination (in the Rorschach sense), discontinuity in thought process, intrusion of illogical material, and the presence of incomprehensible autistic material were some of the features observed.

An example of the emergence of the primary process, an experience which was associated with feelings of unreality, can be found in the following:

> I had odd thoughts . . . concerning the house number (which I live at now) and where I used to live. . . . Something about not being sure and being confused as to past experiences (and present ones), past locations . . . when I was a child. . . .

Unusual forgetfulness and many parapraxes were part of the disturbances by primary process material. At times, associations were so "free" that it was very difficult to follow the story the patient meant to relate. The difficulty of following the patient's story seemed to lend itself particularly well to rating—an overall view of just how much interference there was with communication in a particular hour.

Ratings of anxiety and depression leaned heavily upon the Elmhurst Scale used in a previous study of drug effects (*4*).

Medication Treatment Schedule and Administration

At the end of the initial interview (just prior to the beginning of the study proper), the patient was given a bottle of capsules, instructed to take three capsules per day, and to return the bottle at the next interview. At the end of the subsequent meeting she was given a second bottle of identically appearing capsules with the same instructions. This procedure was repeated until a total of ten bottles were thus received and returned by the patient. Each capsule in a given bottle contained either chlordiazepoxide (10 mg. per capsule) or placebos, identical in appearance to those of the chlordiazepoxide. At the end of the study, the set of ratings pertaining to a given interview was then related to the medication the patient was on during the week's period immediately preceding the interview, providing a basis for the comparison between effects on chlordiazepoxide and those on placebo. The actual sequence of medication corresponding to each psychotherapy session was as indicated in Table 1.

It should be noted that the therapist was not aware of the medication the patient was on during a given week, nor did he know the points at which a change in medication was made.

Distinguishing between Possible Effects of Psychotherapy and Differences in Effect between Medications

The purpose of the methodology described in this paper is the evaluation, based on observations made during the course of psychotherapy, of the comparative efficacy of two medications. The purpose was, of course, not that of evaluating the effect of the psychotherapy itself. Nevertheless in the analysis of the data one must take into consideration the possible effect of psychotherapy (confounded with the effect of time) as a factor in in-

TABLE 1

Medication Sequence

Session No.	Medication
0*	None
1	Placebo
2	Chlordiazepoxide
3	Chlordiazepoxide
4	Chlordiazepoxide
5	Placebo
6	Placebo
7	Placebo
8	Chlordiazepoxide
9	Chlordiazepoxide
10	Chlordiazepoxide

* The initial interview.

fluencing levels of psychopathology as distinct from the influence of differential drug effects. For this reason one cannot, say, simply divide the time-span into consecutive halves with one medication scheduled for the entire first-half, and the other for the second. Such a procedure would then obviously confound differential drug effects with those of psychotherapy and of time. In using the intensive design for the evaluation of differential effect between two medications, one must, therefore, utilize a design which allows for a number of alternations back and forth between the medications throughout the course of the study. An elementary statistical approach to the analysis of data thus obtained is suggested in Figure 1. Here, as an example, the sequence of evidence of primary process ratings is plotted along the time axis (connecting consecutive points, and identifying each plotted point according to whether the observation to which it corresponds was made following a week of placebo or after a week on chlordiazepoxide). A next step is to fit a trend line to the data. Finally, we study and analyze the configuration of plotted points and their identifying medication in relation to their position with respect to the fitted trend line.

It may be of some interest to view the data plotted in Figure 1 from a descriptive point of view before presenting the results of any formal statistical analysis. First, it is noted that over the

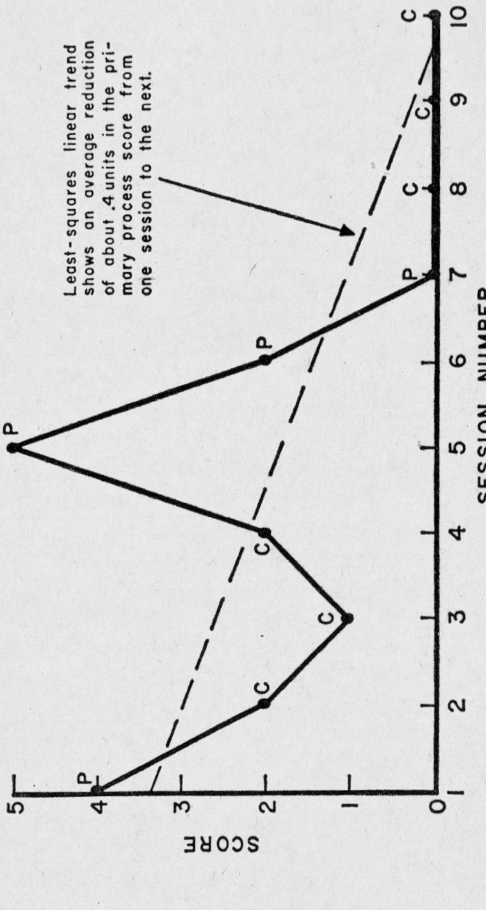

Fig. 1. Sequence of primary process ratings.

ten weeks of the combined administration of psychotherapy and medication (the latter in accordance with the schedule given in Table 1) the fitted trend line describes an *average* decline in the primary process pathology score, of about .4 units per week (*i.e.*, from one session's rating to the next). We note further, that three of the four observations which follow a week of placebo definitely lie above the trend line, indicating a worse-than-average score, while five of the six points relating to the use of chlordiazepoxide are below the trend line, indicating a better-than-average score.[1]

Table 2 presents a tabular analysis of the primary process ratings, comparing averages on chlordiazepoxide with those on placebo. These comparisons are made using both the trend-adjusted scores and the raw scores. Averages over the entire run are compared between active medication and placebo, as well as averages based on subsequences of observations on the same medication. It is seen that the difference in the average scores favor the active medication over the placebo, and that in this particular set of data the use of the trend-adjusted score reduces the difference from that obtained by the corresponding raw score averages by a small fraction. We also note that in going from one subsequence to the next, on the two occasions when the alternation went from placebo to chlordiazepoxide, the average primary process score dropped while the cases in which the direction was from chlordiazepoxide to placebo the average increased. Further, primary process averages for each of the two subsequences on chlordiazepoxide are distinctly below each average on placebo in both the raw and trend-adjusted sequences.

In considering the data plotted in Figure 1, one notes a zero score on placebo at the seventh week followed by three consecutive weeks of zeros on chlordiazepoxide. One might raise the question as to whether the patient had not improved to the point

[1] It should be noted that the singular observation on chlordiazepoxide which lies above the trend line is the last in the series, and it has an actual primary process pathology score of zero (which was also true of the last four observations). Thus its representation as worse-than-average, or rather worse-than-trend, is in this case the result of having selected a straight line trend for reasons of simplicity of exposition. A somewhat more complex trend fitted to the data could have eliminated this feature, perhaps adding slightly to the favorable comparison between active medication and placebo.

TABLE 2

Evidence of Primary Process

Session No.	Medication	Raw Scores		Trend-Adjusted Scores	
		Session Score	Sequence Average	Session Score	Sequence Average
0	None	5	5.0	—	—
1	Placebo	4	4.0	2.2	2.2
2	Chlordiazepoxide	2		0.6	
3	Chlordiazepoxide	1	1.7	0.0	0.7
4	Chlordiazepoxide	2		1.4	
5	Placebo	5		4.8	
6	Placebo	2	2.3	2.2	2.5
7	Placebo	0		0.6	
8	Chlordiazepoxide	0		0.9	
9	Chlordiazepoxide	0	0.0	1.3	1.3
10	Chlordiazepoxide	0		1.7	
Placebo mean		2.75		2.45	
Chlordiazepoxide mean		0.83		0.98	

of being free of the symptom by the end of the seventh week, thus invalidating for purposes of comparison the subsequent three zeros on the active medication. A counter-argument might then be in the form of an assertion that while the patient first finally achieved a zero score on placebo, it is not unlikely that three consecutive weeks on chlordiazepoxide helped keep her there. Reference to Table 2 shows that taking trend into account has the effect of adjusting the last few scores upward in the manner of a compromise. An element of clinical judgment, with regard to the dynamics of the particular case, insofar as this may be related to the stability of so rapid a leveling in the rating independently of the medication, would appear to be unavoidable in such an instance. A longer sequence of observations which would have included a few more alternations between the active and inert medications might have obviated the need for heavy reliance on such a judgment. This is, of course, related to the point made earlier about shortcomings inherent in small samples, whether dealing with a small time-sample of the individual case in the intensive design, or with small numbers of patients in testing between groups in the more conventional extensive design.

Summary of Results on Other Items

As was the case in the ratings on *evidence of primary process,* the weekly observations on each of the other variables, namely, *anxiety, confusion, hostility, "sexual flooding," depersonalization,* and *ability to communicate,* each had more favorable averages on chlordiazepoxide than on placebo. Table 3 shows a compari-

TABLE 3

Effects: Raw and Trend-Adjusted Scores

	Average Raw Scores		Average Trend-Adjusted Scores	
	Chlordiazepoxide	Placebo	Chlordiazepoxide	Placebo
Primary process	0.83	2.75	0.98	2.45
Anxiety	0.75	1.75	1.40	2.15
Confusion	0.67	2.00	1.37	2.40
Hostility	0.83	1.50	1.63	2.05
"Sexual flooding"	0.83	1.75	0.98	1.45
Depersonalization	0.67	2.75	1.45	3.32
Ability to communicate	0.50*	1.75*	0.35*	1.37*
Depression	1.00	1.25	†	†

* The lower the numerical score, the better the ability to communicate.

† Depression is the only item for which a decreasing trend was not at all evident from the data.

son between effects, both within the raw scores and the trend-adjusted scores on each of the observed outcome variables.

In discussing the primary process ratings given in Table 2, it was noted that with respect to both the raw and the trend-adjusted scores, alternations from a subsequence of observations on placebo to a subsequence on chlordiazepoxide corresponded to an improvement in the average rating for a subsequence, while an alternation in the opposite direction (*i.e.*, from chlordiazepoxide to placebo) resulted in a worsening, *i.e.*, in an increase in corresponding average primary process pathology. Among the other seven observed items of psychopathology similar fluctuations in subsequence-averages occurred in *anxiety, confusion, depersonalization,* and *ability to communicate*. This did not hold for the trend-adjusted scores in "*sexual flooding*" nor for the raw scores in *hostility*. While this type of alternation in sequence averages also appeared in the raw scores on *depression,* very little significance can be attached to this because of the relatively small difference between placebo and chlordiazepoxide in the overall average rating for *depression*. (See Table 3.)

Statistical Analysis and Questions of Statistical Significance

Given a set of results showing differences between two medications, it is no longer merely the avant-garde who have learned to ask the question: "Are the results statistically significant?" or "What is the level of significance in the difference between drug effects?" Anyone who has had the least exposure to clinical research is aware of the operation of the laws of chance, and of the problem of differentiating between true effects and chance effects. However, what is not always clearly understood is that there is no absolute or unambiguous answer to a question concerning an exact level of significance *without reference to some mathematical statistical model* which for purposes of statistical inference must be assumed to be correct if probability statements such as those concerning levels of significance are to remain credible. The normal distribution, and the mathematically related Student-*t* and the chi-square distributions, for example, are mathematical models whose absolute truth in relation to a set of data can never be demonstrated. They can only be assumed to be reasonable models of the reality (sometimes also assumed) to which they are applied. This is, of course, not intended in any way as an argument against the use of the normal and related distributions. There is certainly much empirical evidence to support its use in very many diverse areas, and the central limit theorem of statistics, better known to statisticians than to clinicians, adds a theoretical argument in favor of its use. Nevertheless it is, say, by no means always clear, as to whether a given set of data ought to be analyzed by the use of tests based on an underlying assumption of normality, or whether a nonparametric approach should be used. The investigator who applies both types of tests to the same set of data will in general obtain two distinct levels of significance. Fortunately, in a great many cases, one such level serves as a fairly good approximation of the other. But when one test yields a level of .04 and the other a level .07, an obsession about reaching "the" .05 level can provide an unfortunate and objectively unnecessary degree of discomfort. The point may be a bit belabored here, but it is made to emphasize that there is generally speaking no single, simple, precise, and unambiguous answer to the question of statistical significance which can be taken as absolute. Judgment, statistical as well as clinical, often has to be invoked with an awareness of one's possible biases.

Another type of problem which relates to the question of how well a statistical model fits the reality of a given clinical design, and one which is often more difficult to handle than the question of parametric versus nonparametric approaches, is that of statistical independence. The question of choosing between a parametric and a nonparametric test is of relatively little consequence if in both cases statistical independence is assumed and the reality of the clinical setting is such that such an assumption may be tenable. It has been suggested (*5, 6*) that the assumption of statistical independence in the observation of individual patients on the same ward (as is generally implicit in statistical tests applied to groups of patients) was open to serious question and could consequently result in gross errors in statistical inference. Data subsequently presented (*9*) provide strong statistical evidence of such lack of statistical independence.

A statistical analysis of the data gathered in this study falls into the area of statistics known as time-series analysis. The question of statistical independence is a matter of concern in the analysis of data from a time-series to the extent that a particular observation may be statistically dependent on the previous observation, or on a sequence of immediately preceding observations. Thus, the level of a patient's pathology during an observation period may be statistically dependent on his level during the previous period *in a given setting or context of observation.* The greater the statistical dependence on previous states, the less is there an immediate justification for, say, a standard application of the *t*-test to determine significant differences between time-series segments. However, unlike the situation in extensive designs in which tests between groups of patients are only performed at a single point in time, or even when an initial point is used as a covariate for adjusting end-point observations, the data from the time-series itself provides information concerning the degree of dependence in the series. If this turns out to be quite small, then standard tests, such as the *t*-test, may be expected to provide reasonably valid significance levels.

Applying a *t*-test to residuals from trend for each of the eight items, the largest *t*-value, 3.117, obtained for *depersonalization,* was significant at the .01 level. A *t*-value of 1.89 was obtained from the *evidence of primary process* residuals, which is significant at the .05 level (one-tailed test). The corresponding *t*-values of each of the other six items were all smaller, and did not reach generally accepted levels of significance. Of these, the one closest to significance was *ability to communicate,* with a single-tailed level of .09. The smallest difference, as noted above, was that obtained for *depression.*

When a *t*-test was applied to the *raw* scores on the items found to be significant on the trend-adjusted scores, acceptable levels of significance were also found. The *t*-value for *evidence of primary process* remained practically unchanged (increasing slightly to 1.90) at the .05 level, while that for *depersonalization* declined from 3.12 to 2.15. The latter value, however, is still significant at a (one-tailed) level of about .035. A third and final test for drug effect applied to the *primary process and depersonalization* ratings involved a covariance analysis in which time (*i.e.,* research hour number) was taken as the covariate as a means of adjusting for trend. In this test, the significance level for both variables dropped somewhat, falling between .05 and .06.

The question as to which of the three procedures used in testing for true drug effect is the most valid can only be answered theoretically, and in terms of which of the corresponding statistical models is the most valid. This is not always a facile decision, particularly when so small a series of observations is involved. One might ask whether adjustment for trend is valid for this set of data, as the trend line itself was not particularly marked in relation to the variation of the data about the trend line. On the basis of so small a set of observations, this may still be a matter of judgment.

In the analysis of covariance as it has been applied here, the assumption was implicit that two parallel linear trends existed, one corresponding to the placebo and the other to chlordiazepoxide. The analysis of covariance then tested the null hypothesis that the lines are identical.

Analyzing the residuals from the single trend line (corresponding to Figure 1) as was first done does not necessarily test directly or make any direct assumption about two separate trends, but rather tests for a significant difference in departures from a common trend.

Intensive Design in Relation to Placebo Reaction, Follow-up, and Subsequent Treatment of the Individual Case

A particularly valuable property of designs in which one tests *primarily* for significant effects within the individual patient rather than between patients is the specificity of the results—in terms of significance or nonsignificance—in relation to the patient himself. The procedure not only provides valid data for evaluating whether a treatment is effective, but incorporates the feature of identifying particular patient characteristics which may be relevant to the effect of the treatment in accordance with the results provided by the series of data from each patient in such a study. The comparatively large number of hypotheses which one can thus test by applying an intensive design in a relatively few well-selected (not necessarily randomly selected) patients with some variation in their characteristics, makes it possible to develop an organized program of clinical research with more clearly specified objectives than can possibly be achieved in a sequence of extensive designs in which hypotheses can only be tested for groups of patients taken as a whole. This can be achieved by a systematic selection of patients, chosen for similarities and dissimilarities in particular patient characteristics, and in relation to ongoing results provided by sets of intensive studies.

Apart from the rather broad implications for clinical research methodology as such, the use of the intensive design has, as a corollary, a particular use in the subsequent treatment of the individual study-patient himself.

First, consider such questions as, "Is patient A a placebo reactor?" or "Did A actually benefit from the active medication?" Questions such as these cannot be answered as a consequence of patient A's participation in a clinical research project in which hypotheses are tested between groups of patients. For example, in a study in which one group of patients is on an active medication, and the other on placebo and if A belongs to the group selected for treatment on the active medication, and if, further, A should show an improved score, there would be no way of determining from the data of the study whether A improved because he was on an active medication, or whether he merely reacted as he might have to a placebo. If A had instead been selected for treatment with placebo then 1) a failure to improve would give no information concerning how effective treatment with the active medication would have been for him; or 2) if he showed improvement on placebo one still could not state whether improvement might not have been even greater on the active medication. Neither, incidentally, can one state definitively that the reaction would necessarily have been a true placebo effect. Such an effect (*i.e.*, improvement without active medication) can logically result from a complex of circumstances which happened to coincide with the administration of the placebo, or with the point in time at which the placebo observation was made and may have been entirely unrelated to it.

Thus, with respect to the continuing treatment of the individual patient participating in the extensive model, the results of a particular study which may show a statistically significant greater improvement on active medication than on placebo, will not, in general, and with any degree of confidence provide specific information as to whether a *particular* patient benefited on the active medication and therefore might be benefited by its continued use beyond the study. In a very loose way (because of the wide range of various relevant characteristics of patients) all it does is to indicate that the active medication is a better bet than the placebo. Now, if the study involved one active drug against another (instead of against a placebo) even so gross an assessment would be difficult or, perhaps more dangerously misleading, for presumably some of the patients who apparently improved on the drug which came out worse in the comparison might not have been helped by the "better" drug.

Although the use of a crossover within the framework of the extensive model may be a little more informative about the individual case, it would still not be anywhere near adequate from the point of view of statistical significance *within* the individual case. Several crossovers back and forth for each patient would, of course, provide data for intensive model analysis.

In an intensive design, again apart from its broader implications for research, a statistically significant finding is significant, in particular, for a specific patient, and therefore may well indicate the course of further treatment for that patient. The small number of cases that one requires for an application of the intensive model, the minimum number actually being a single case (as in the present study) thus not only allows the practicing psychotherapist to engage in meaningful research to satisfy some of his own interests without requiring elaborate, and/or institutional settings, but also represents a use of research methodology in actual treatment and for the maximum benefit of the patient under treatment.

Clinically, the patient under observation in this study did well. Some months after termination of this series of therapeutic interviews, she had some recurrence of anxiety in response to reality difficulties, at which time a prescription for a short period of medication with chlordiazepoxide seemed efficacious.

SUMMARY

This is an experimental application of intensive design to the evaluation of drug effect during the course of individual psychotherapy. Intensive design represents an approach to clinical research in which observations concerning each patient in a study are made in such a way as to permit the application of statistical methods to the testing of intra-patient hypotheses concerning treatment or other effects. This is in contrast to the more conventional approach to the design of clinical research in which the testing of hypotheses is limited to those concerning groups of patients taken as a whole. In this application of the single-case design, a double-blind technique was applied toward evaluating the possible advantages of the use of drugs as an adjunct to analytically oriented psychotherapy. While the study was essentially one in feasibility, with a rather severe limitation on its length, statistically significant effects favoring chlordiazepoxide over placebo were nevertheless obtained on a number of scale items constructed especially for the patient under study by the psychiatric author, whose observations were recorded at the end of each hour of psychotherapy and subsequently related to the patient's medication during the week preceding the given hour of psychotherapy. The possible usefulness of the results from an intensive design for the continuing treatment of the patient following the completion of the research is also demonstrated.

REFERENCES

1. Bellak, L. The use of oral barbiturates in psychotherapy. *Amer. J. Psychiat., 105,* 849–850, 1949.
2. Bellak, L. Research in psychoanalysis. *Psychoanal. Quart., 30,* 519–548, 1961.
3. Bellak, L. and Smith, M. B. An experimental exploration of the psychoanalytic process. *Psychoanal. Quart., 25,* 385–414, 1956.
4. Bellak, L., Salk, L. and Rosenhan, D. A process study of the effects of Deprol on depression. *J. Nerv. Ment. Dis., 132,* 531–538, 1961.
5. Chassan, J. B. Statistical inference and the single case in clinical design. *Psychiatry, 23,* 173–184, 1960.
6. Chassan, J. B. Stochastic models of the single case as the basis of clinical research design. *Behavioral Sci., 6,* 42–50, 1961.
7. Chassan, J. B. On the unreliability of reliability and some other consequences of the assumption of probabilistic patient-states. *Psychiatry, 20,* 163–171, 1957.
8. Chassan, J. B. On the development of clinical statistical systems for psychiatry. *Biometrics, 15,* 396–404, 1959.
9. Kellam, S. and Chassan, J. B. Social context and system fluctuation. *Psychiatry, 25,* 370–381, 1962.

* Note

By the Editors of the Series

In the field of psychology we believe that the student ought to get the "feel" of experimentation by reading original source materials. In this way he can acquire a better understanding of the discipline by seeing scientific ideas grow and change. However, one of the main problems in teaching is the limited availability of these sources, which communicate most effectively the personality of the author and the excitement of ongoing research.

For these reasons we have decided to edit several books,* each devoted to a particular problem in psychology. In every case we attempt to select problems that have been and are controversial—that have been and still are alive. We intend to present these problems as a set of selected original articles, arranged in historical order and in order of progress in the field. We believe that it is important for the student to see that theories and researches build on what has gone before; that one study leads to another, that theory leads to research and then to revision of theory. We believe that *telling* the student this does not make the same kind of impression as letting him see it happen in actuality. The idea is for the student to read and build ideas for himself.

Suggestions for Use—These readings books can be used by the student in either of two ways. They are organized so that, with the help of the instructor (or of the students if used in seminars), a topic can be covered at length and in depth. This would necessitate lectures or discussions on articles not covered in the series to fill in the gaps. On the other hand, each book taken alone will give a student a good idea of the problem being covered and its historical background as well as its present state and the direction it seems to be taking.

* (Pub. note: a sub-series within the Insight Book Series.)

VAN NOSTRAND INSIGHT BOOKS

PSYCHOLOGY N9896

About this book:

Clincial psychology has been one of the few areas of psychology where good examples of the application of experimental procedures have not been readily available. This collection of fifteen articles illustrates various approaches to the experimental investigation of the single case. Although the studies presented differ in their theoretical orientation, the methods they use, the degree of experimental sophistication involved, and the extent of their success, they all represent tentative bridges between the experimentalist and the clinician. The value of these methods for both the assessment and modification of behavior is demonstrated, and the rationale of such approaches and some simple statistical procedures that may be used are discussed in three introductory articles. Students and instructors will find *N=1* to be a valuable source book, as will all mental health workers in light of the immediate relevance of the methods in the clinical area.

VAN NOSTRAND INSIGHT BOOKS

Insight Books are devoted to filling a vital need in the efficient study of human behavior. By making available, in paperback, essential materials that are frequently inaccessible or often neglected in a more expensive form, the Insight Series renders a valuable service to students, teachers, and interested laymen. Drawn from psychology and its allied fields, the bulk of the books published will deal with the following categories: 1) studies of enduring problems in psychology through original sources; 2) selections from their own works by contemporary behavioral scientists; and 3) authoritative discussions of timely, even controversial, issues.

DAVID C. McCLELLAND is general editor of Insight Books. Currently Professor of Psychology in the Department of Social Relations at Harvard University, he is also an established author in experimental and theoretical psychology. Among his recent books is *The Achieving Society*, published by Van Nostrand.

Along with Dr. McClelland, Dr. Robert C. Birney of Hampshire College